HALL AND COLMAN'S
DISEASES OF THE EAR, NOSE AND THROAT

Commissioning Editors: Laurence Hunter & Michael Parkinson
Project Editor: Sarah Keer-Keer
Project Controller: Frances Affleck
Designer: Erik Bigland

HALL AND COLMAN'S
DISEASES OF THE EAR, NOSE AND THROAT

EDITED BY

Martin Burton
Consultant Otolaryngologist
The Radcliffe Infirmary, Oxford

FIFTEENTH EDITION

WITH CO-AUTHORS:

Susanna Leighton
Consultant Otolaryngologist
Department of Paediatric Otolaryngology
Great Ormond Street Hospital, London

Andrew Robson
Consultant Otolaryngologist
City General Hospital, Carlisle

John Russell
Consultant Otolaryngologist,
Mater Misericordiae Hospital, Dublin

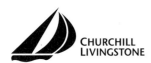
CHURCHILL
LIVINGSTONE

EDINBURGH LONDON NEW YORK OXFORD PHILADELPHIA ST LOUIS SYDNEY TORONTO 2000

CHURCHILL LIVINGSTONE
An imprint of Elsevier Limited

First Edition 1937   Ninth Edition 1969
Second Edition 1941   Tenth edition 1973
Third Edition 1944   Eleventh edition 1975
Fourth Edition 1948   Twelfth edition 1981
Fifth Edition 1952   Thirteenth edition 1987
Sixth Edition 1956   Fourteenth edition 1992
Seventh edition 1959   Fifteenth edition 2000
Eighth edition 1967

ISBN 0 443 06190 4
    Reprinted 2000, 2001, 2003, 2006

International Student Edition 0 443 07019 9
    Reprinted 2000

British Library Cataloguing in Publication Data
A catalogue record for this book is available from the British
Library

Library of Congress Cataloguing in Publication Data
A catalogue record for this book is available from the Library of
Congress

Medical knowledge is constantly changing. As new information
becomes available, changes in treatment, procedures, equipment
and the use of drugs become necessary. The editors, contributor
and the publishers have taken care to ensure that the information
given in this text is accurate and up to date. However, readers are
strongly advised to confirm that the information, especially with
regard to drug usage, complies with the latest legislation and
standards of practice.

ELSEVIER your source for books,
journals and multimedia
in the health sciences
www.elsevierhealth.com

Working together to grow
libraries in developing countries
www.elsevier.com | www.bookaid.org | www.sabre.org

ELSEVIER   BOOK AID International   Sabre Foundation

Printed in China
B/06/02

The
publisher's
policy is to use
**paper manufactured
from sustainable forests**

Contents

Section 4
The mouth and salivary glands

Section 5
The larynx, pharynx and oesophagus

Preface

This is the fifteenth edition of what has become a classic text but the first to have been revised and, in part, re-written by a new team. In taking over from Bernard Colman, the contributors are in no doubt that this book is still very much 'Hall and Colman'. We all worked for Bernard Colman as registrars or senior house officers and are indebted to him for much that we learned. It is perhaps a measure of the breadth of his talents, and the super-specialised nature of our own, that a multi-author team was needed for this edition.

We have tried to keep the popular style of previous editions. The book is aimed at generalists – both general practitioners and surgical trainees at the beginning of their training – and the enquiring medical student. Equally, we hope it will provide a broad introduction to the new trainee in otolaryngology – head & neck surgery. Some diseases that are described are now rare in the United Kingdom. We are mindful of the fact that those working elsewhere in the world have often found the book useful.

As always, we are grateful to our colleagues who kindly provided illustrations and photographs. We particularly acknowledge Mr Rogan Corbridge, Dr Philip Anslow, Nobel Biocare and Cochlear. We thank Sarah Keer-Keer and Jim Killgore of Harcourt Brace, who patiently steered us through the production process, and Mr Nick Murrant, Consultant Otolaryngologist Carlisle, for advice on parts of the text. We also thank the Medical Illustration Departments of Carlisle Hospitals NHS Trust and City Hospitals, Sunderland and Great Ormond Street Hospital for Children NHS Trust. Finally, but certainly not least, our families gave us the time and encouragement we all needed to undertake this project; to them our most grateful thanks.

Oxford, 1999
MJB

THE EAR 1

Anatomy and physiology of the ear

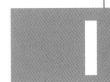

ANATOMY

The external ear

The external ear comprises the pinna and the external auditory meatus. The outer third is cartilaginous, the inner two-thirds are bony.

The pinna is composed of cartilage covered with perichondrium, to which the skin and superficial tissues are very closely bound. The cartilaginous meatus is similarly constructed, containing in addition hair follicles and ceruminous glands which secrete wax. The hair follicles are confined to the most lateral part of the meatus. Owing to the tight union of cartilage and skin any inflammatory process (such as a boil in the cartilaginous part of the meatus) can be extremely painful.

The epithelium lining the bony meatus is much thinner and devoid of those integuments that characterise the thicker skin of the cartilaginous canal. The epithelial lining is contiguous with the eardrum as a single layer of stratified epithelium.

The external meatus varies in size and form with growth. There are considerable variations among individuals. In the adult there is an angle in the meatus: the outer part runs upwards and backwards as it passes inwards; the inner part runs more horizontally. Accordingly, the pinna must be pulled upwards and backwards when using a speculum to examine the eardrum. In children, on the other hand, the meatus is shorter and straighter and the drum can often be examined without this manoeuvre.

The tympanic membrane

The tympanic membrane, or eardrum, consists of three layers: an outer epithelial layer, a middle layer of fibrous tissue and an inner layer of mucous membrane. The eardrum is supported around its periphery by a fibrous thickening, the annulus. This fibrous annulus fits in turn into a slot in the tympanic bone, which develops separately from the body of the petrous bone, but is eventually incorporated in it. There is a small deficiency superiorly, known as the notch of Rivinus. The fibrous annulus is also deficient in this small portion of the upper part of its circumference.

The drum membrane is divided into two parts: the pars tensa and the pars flaccida. In the latter the middle layer is comprised of irregular elastic fibres, hence the flaccidity. This part of the drum is small and comprises the uppermost part occupying the notch of Rivinus. It is sometimes difficult to see. It is frequently referred to as the 'attic'. Perforations in this area are potentially unsafe, as will be seen later.

Landmarks of the eardrum

The most prominent landmark is the handle of the malleus, seen as a white streak running from anterosuperiorly down to the approximate centre of the drum. At its upper end is a small projection – the lateral process of the malleus.

In the drum membrane are two folds running anteriorly and posteriorly from the lateral process. These are the anterior and posterior mallear folds.

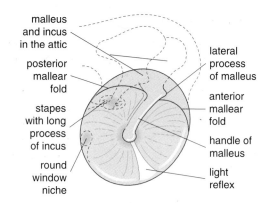

Fig. 1.1 The right eardrum. The broken lines indicate the relationships of the middle ear structures.

The part of the drum above these folds is the pars flaccida (Fig. 1.1).

The middle ear

The middle ear cleft comprises the middle ear, the eustachian tube, the mastoid antrum and cells, and may be divided into three. The uppermost portion is the attic or *epi*tympanum, the middle the *meso*-tympanum and the lowest the *hypo*tympanum. The attic is that part of the middle ear above the level of the mallear folds. It is divided into a number of small pockets by parts of the ossicles, their ligaments and mucosal folds. Chronic infection may localise in these spaces. Note that the middle ear extends beyond the limits of the drum (Figs 1.2 and 1.3).

The anterior wall of the middle ear has an opening low down in the wall. This is the opening of the eustachian tube. Above it is the canal for the tensor tympani muscle.

There are several important structures on the medial wall, most of which is occupied by a rounded swelling known as the promontory. This is the bony covering of the basal turn of the cochlea. Running approximately horizontally superior to it is the facial nerve, covered by a thin layer of bone. Posteroinferior to the promontory is a deep recess known as the round window niche. The round window itself is closed by a thin membrane, deep to which is the scala tympani of the cochlea. Posterosuperior to the promontory is a somewhat similar opening which is occupied by the footplate

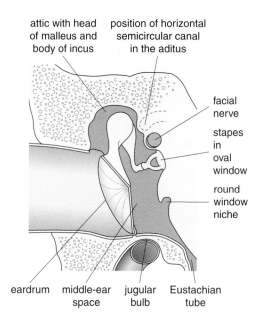

Fig. 1.2 Coronal section of middle ear.

of the stapes bone and leads into the scala vestibuli of the cochlea.

The posterior wall contains an opening (the aditus) high up, which leads to the mastoid antrum. In the floor of the entrance to the aditus there is a smooth swelling that is caused by the bony horizontal semicircular canal of the labyrinth. Just below the entrance to the aditus is a small pyramid of bone which contains the stapedius muscle.

Below the floor of the middle ear lies the jugular bulb; superior to the middle ear is the dura mater of the middle cranial fossa. Both are usually covered by thin bone.

The middle ear is an air-containing space with three ossicles: the malleus, incus and stapes. The handle of the malleus is firmly embedded in the middle layer of the drum and its head articulates in the attic with the body of the incus. The incus has two processes: the short process is attached to the lip of the aditus; the long process descends to articulate with the head of the stapes. The stapes resembles a stirrup and its footplate occupies the oval window. It is attached at the margin by the annular ligament, forming a simple fibrous joint – the stapediovestibular joint. The malleoincudal and incudostapedial joints are synovial.

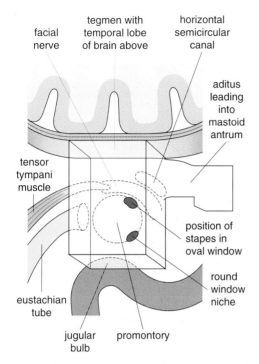

facial nerve

tegmen with temporal lobe of brain above

horizontal semicircular canal

aditus leading into mastoid antrum

tensor tympani muscle

position of stapes in oval window

round window niche

eustachian tube

jugular bulb

promontory

Fig. 1.3 Schematic view of left middle ear and its relations.

Muscles of the middle ear

There are two muscles in the middle ear: the tensor tympani inserted into the neck of the malleus; and the stapedius inserted into the neck of the stapes. The latter contracts reflexly in response to loud noise. The effect is to restrict the vibration of the drum and ossicular chain by increasing their tension and stiffness. The sensitivity of the ear is thus reduced and delicate structures of the cochlea are protected from damage.

The mastoid air spaces

The mastoid antrum is the largest and most constant of the air spaces within the mastoid bone, and indeed may be the only air space. Most mastoids, however, are pneumatised to some extent, and some are pneumatised very extensively indeed. At first glance the cells may appear to be arranged in a totally haphazard fashion, but in fact they are in well-defined groups that must be sought out individually during a mastoid operation.

Eustachian tube

The eustachian tube communicates with the nasopharynx and has a bony upper portion and cartilaginous lower portion. It is potentially patent and is opened by swallowing. The function of the eustachian tube is to maintain the pressure of air inside the middle ear and mastoid system approximately equal to the external atmospheric pressure. If the middle ear pressure drops, the level of hearing also falls.

The inner ear

The inner ear, or labyrinth, consists of a bony capsule that is almost embedded in the petrous bone (Fig. 1.4). Within this 'otic capsule' is the membranous labyrinth. The otic capsule consists of three parts: anteriorly, the snail-like cochlea; in the middle, the vestibule; and posteriorly, three semicircular canals (Fig. 1.5). The otic capsule is hollow and contains perilymph. Suspended in the perilymph by delicate filamentous strands is the membranous labyrinth. This is a complex series of sacs and tubes containing a different fluid, the endolymph.

The membranous labyrinth consists of several parts (Fig. 1.6). The three membranous semicircular canals (horizontal, anterior and posterior) occupy the corresponding bony canals and are set at right angles to each other, each representing a plane in space. The two vertical canals – the anterior and posterior – unite posteromedially, forming a shared channel, the common crus. The anterior end of each canal is dilated to form its ampulla, and this region contains a patch of neuroepithelium called the crista. Tiny hairs arising from the crista are embedded in the overlying gelatinous cupola. This is displaced when endolymph moves within the canal. The normal stimulus that excites the ampullary nerve is angular acceleration, but in clinical testing convection currents produced by hot or cold caloric stimulation can be used.

The three anterior ends of the canals, the common crus and the posterior end of the horizontal canal all open into the utricle. This, and the saccule, lie in the central part of the membranous labyrinth, within the vestibule of the bony labyrinth. Each possesses a patch of neuroepithelium known as the

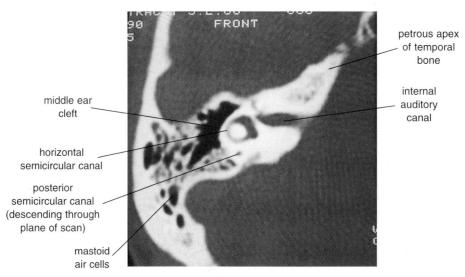

Fig. 1.4 CT scan of temporal bone in axial plane. (1) internal auditory meatus; (2) vestibule; (3) horizontal semicircular canal; (4) posterior semicircular canal; (5) sigmoid sinus.

macula. This resembles the ampullary crista, except that the overlying membrane is flatter and contains particles of calcium carbonate called otoliths. Gravitational pull and linear acceleration stimulate the macula of the utricle and saccule. The utricle and saccule are joined by the Y-shaped endolymphatic duct, the long stem of which extends to the endolymphatic sac. This sac lies between the two layers of dura on the posterior surface of the petrous bone, i.e. in the posterior cranial fossa. In humans, the sac is probably concerned with absorption of endolymph.

The membranous cochlear duct is a simple tube situated in the bony cochlea and coiled for two and a half turns around its central bony modiolus. Its small connection to the saccule is called the ductus reuniens.

When seen in the bisected bony cochlea, the cochlear duct appears triangular in cross-section in each turn (Fig. 1.7). Reissner's membrane, the stria

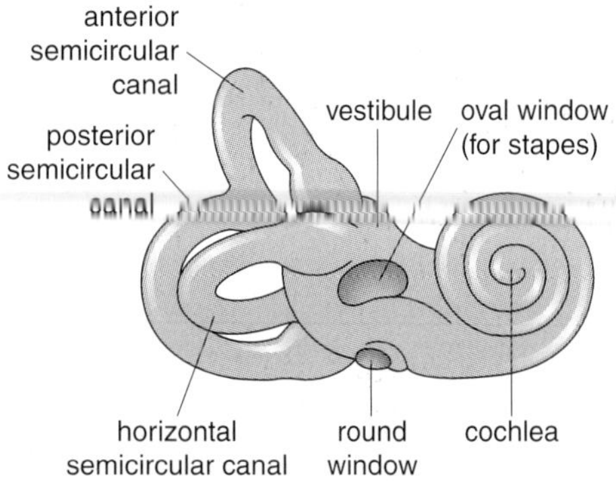

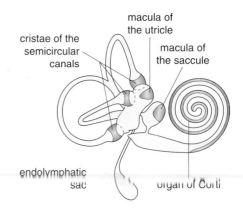

Fig. 1.6 Lateral view of right membranous labyrinth, which is contained within the bony labyrinth, floating in the perilymph. Sensory epithelium is located in the crista of each semicircular canal and the macula of the utricle and saccule. The strip of sensory epithelium in the cochlea is the organ of Corti. The endolymphatic sac lies on the posterior surface of the temporal bone.

Fig. 1.5 Right bony labyrinth (lateral view).

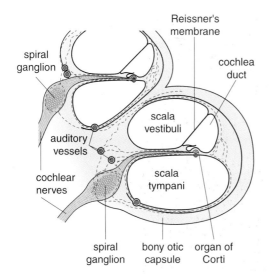

Fig. 1.7 Section through cochlea.

pani on its inferior side. In the lower (basal) turn of the cochlea these two scala end at the oval and round windows respectively but at the apex they are continuous with each other around the end of the cochlear duct. The scala tympani connects with the subarachnoid space, to which infection can spread from the labyrinth.

The neuroepithelium of the cochlea is arranged as a ribbon along the entire length of the basilar membrane and is known as the organ of Corti (Fig. 1.8). The particular part activated by a sound depends on the frequency, high frequencies being represented at the base of the cochlea, low frequencies at the apex. Nerve fibres from the organ of Corti pass centrally as the cochlear nerve. This also contains efferent fibres from the brainstem to the cochlea – the olivocochlear bundle.

The ampullary, utricular and saccular nerves unite to form the vestibular nerve, the ganglion of which lies in the internal auditory meatus (Fig. 1.9). The spiral ganglion of the cochlear nerve is situated in the modiolus in the centre of the cochlea itself.

vascularis and the basilar membrane form its three sides. The cochlear duct is so situated that it is bathed by perilymph on two sides: the scala vestibuli on its superior aspect and the scala tym-

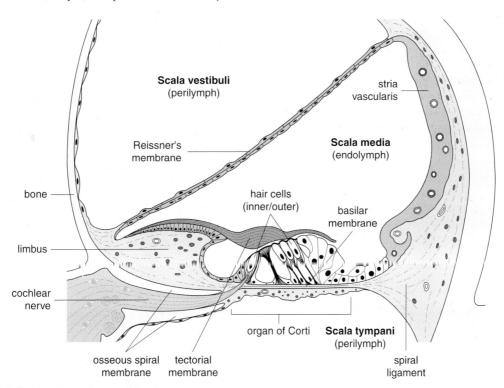

Fig. 1.8 Cochlear duct and organ of Corti.

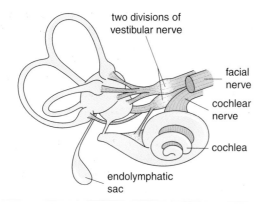

Fig. 1.9 Innervation of cochlear and vestibular system.

PHYSIOLOGY

Middle ear mechanism

To achieve successful stimulation of the cochlea via the middle ear it is essential that a sound pressure difference is present between the oval and round windows. In the normal ear this is obtained by the preferential transmission of vibration through the drum and the ossicular chain. Comparatively little sound travels direct to the round window; indeed, the presence of the drum itself provides for its sound protection.

Although the ossicular chain provides certain acoustic advantages and is a highly efficient part of the sound transformer mechanism of the middle ear, a simple columella is compatible with relatively good hearing. This is the principle of certain types of tympanoplasty.

Good hearing can indeed be obtained without an ossicular chain as long as there are two mobile windows and sound protection for one is provided, for example by the remains of the drum. Some tympanoplasty operations depend on this mechanism.

Interruption of the ossicular chain or total loss of the drum results in severe hearing loss, largely because there is no difference in the pressure of sound reaching the two windows.

Reference has already been made to the action of the middle ear muscles (p. 5).

Cochlear mechanism

The cochlea can be stimulated directly by bone conduction as well as by sound passing through the middle ear. It is generally agreed that sound waves are analysed in the cochlea and that each frequency has its own place on the basilar membrane. Ample evidence supports these place theories, with the higher frequencies being represented in the basal part of the cochlea and the lower frequencies in the apex. Helmholtz looked upon the basilar membrane as a simple resonator, but it has long been recognised that the mechanism is far more complicated than this.

Complex mechanical experiments as well as observation of the basilar membrane in action by the Nobel prize-winner von Békésy resulted in his travelling-wave theory. He was able to show that vibration introduced into the oval window of his models resulted in a wave travelling up the basilar membrane, increasing in amplitude as it moved, and finally dying away. The point of maximum amplitude was determined by the frequency introduced, and occurred at a corresponding distance along the basilar membrane. It is now known that the vibration of the basilar membrane is boosted by an active mechanical amplifier mechanism.

Movement of the basilar membrane results in deflection of the stereocilia of the hair cells. The stretching of 'tip links' connecting the stereocilia results in the opening of ion channels in the cell membrane and release of neurotransmitter at the base of the cell. Most of the afferent auditory nerve fibres are stimulated in this way by inner hair cell activity. The outer hair cells play a role in the active mechanical amplifier mechanism. At low frequencies auditory nerve fibres are stimulated in synchrony with the stimulating tone; this is temporal coding. Place coding refers to the process by which stimulation of different parts of the basilar membrane results in activation of different populations of nerve fibres. The role of the olivocochlear bundle is still uncertain but may be related to the active mechanical amplifier mechanism.

Vestibular mechanism

The vestibular system is important in maintaining normal balance. Angular acceleration is detected by the semicircular canals, and linear acceleration and tilt by the saccule and utricle. Deflection of the stereocilia of the hair cells within these organs leads to a change in the resting neural activity of the vestibular nerve fibres.

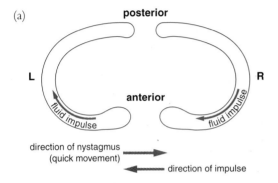

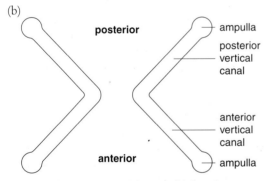

Fig. 1.10 (a) Horizontal canal function. (b) Complementary character of vertically placed anterior and posterior semicircular canals.

The semicircular canals are stimulated by endolymph flow within the lumen, the result of inertial lag of the endolymph at the start and finish of head movement around an axis of rotation. The three canals of one labyrinth are arranged at right angles to each other (Fig. 1.10) and it follows that each canal has a counterpart on the opposite side in the same plane. Movement in any plane may thus be detected. Peripheral vestibular stimulation affects the vestibulo-ocular, vestibulospinal and vestibulo-collic reflexes. Vestibular information is integrated with other inputs to the central nervous system – most importantly from the proprioceptive system (muscle, tendon and joint and skin pressure sensors) and visual system. In this way normal balance is maintained. Information arriving centrally from these different sources is normally in agreement, allowing the body to maintain a high degree of equilibrium. False information fed in by any of the end organs, or dysfunction of the central pathways, will result in some form of dysequilibrium.

> ➤ **Key points**
>
> ➤ Understanding middle ear anatomy is important for interpreting findings on otoscopic examination.
> ➤ The facial nerve passes through the middle ear.
> ➤ Middle ear complications and mastoid problems may be predicted from a knowledge of the relationships of the middle ear and mastoid.

Examination and assessment of the ear

2

EXAMINATION OF THE EAR

When examining the ears, the position of both patient and examiner is important. The patient faces the examiner and the bull's-eye lamp is placed a little behind the patient, level with the left ear. The examiner sits close alongside or in front of the patient, within easy reach for manipulation of the head. The light from the mirror is then focused upon the patient's ear. The smallest and brightest spot of light should be obtained.

The examination begins with inspection of the pinna, and a glance behind the ear may reveal a scar from an operation that the patient had forgotten to mention. Attention is next directed to the external auditory canal.

It used to be standard practice to examine the external canal and tympanic membrane as follows: in examination of the patient's left ear the patient's head is turned slightly to the right or, if the patient is in a movable chair, the chair can be rotated a little to the right. The left hand of the examiner grasps the upper part of the pinna, the pinna being held between the second and third or the third and fourth fingers. The speculum is placed in the external meatus with the right hand and is then taken between the thumb and first finger of the left hand so that the right hand is left free for mopping secretions or removal of wax, for instance.

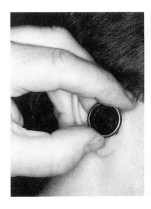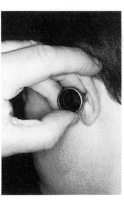

Fig. 2.1 Method of examining the ear holding a speculum and retracting the pinna with the same hand.

The object of this grasp of the pinna is to enable sufficient traction to be put upon the cartilaginous meatus to draw it backwards and upwards to straighten out the angle of the meatus (Fig. 2.1).

With this gentle traction upwards and backwards the drum should be brought into view without trouble. One of the chief difficulties in examining the external meatus is ensuring that the light is focused in the proper direction. It must be directed forwards and upwards, and in some cases the patient's head may almost have to be turned away from the examiner in order to be able to expose the

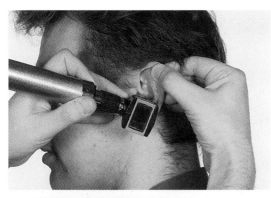

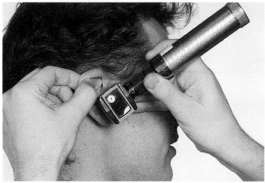

Fig. 2.2 Method of examining the ear using an otoscope and retracting the pinna with the opposite hand.

drum. If the speculum is held properly and the patient's head is at the correct angle, the examiner should be looking at the eardrum.

Nowadays the external canal and eardrum are more usually examined using an otoscope. This is held like a pen (Fig. 2.2), in the right hand for the right ear, left hand for the left. The opposite hand retracts the pinna, as described. The little and ring fingers of the hand holding the otoscope should rest against the side of the patient's head. In this way the instrument is 'fixed' relative to the head and any sudden movement of the examiner's arm will not result in the speculum of the otoscope being driven into the ear canal.

Whichever method of examination is used, the identification of the drum is made partly on the basis of colour, which should be pearly grey. It is lustrous and reflects light. The light reflex takes the shape of a cone, passing from the centre forwards and downwards (Fig. 1.1).

Certain landmarks must be sought in order to identify the drum – the most obvious is the handle of the malleus. At its upper end the lateral process stands out as a small white knob, and from this point the anterior and posterior mallear folds may be identified: the pars flaccida is above, the pars tensa below.

The drum lies at an angle to the observer. The upper posterior part is the nearest and the anterior inferior part the furthest away. The angle in individuals varies considerably, but all the structures noted above are seen at an angle. A view of the anterior part of the eardrum is sometimes limited by the bony hump overlying the temporomandibular joint.

Once the drum is identified, any deviation from normal must be noted, for example colour, retraction or fullness, increased vascularity, scars or perforations. It is also important to observe movement when using the pneumatic attachment to the otoscope. At this stage it is convenient to examine eustachian tube patency by watching for drum movement when the patient autoinflates (p. 13); Not everyone can perform this manoeuvre, however, so failure does not necessarily indicate tubal occlusion.

If the drum cannot be seen, the examiner must not be satisfied until the reason for failure has been found. It may be that the light is not properly directed, the result of which will be that only the posterior wall of the meatus is illuminated.

Any discharge must be carefully traced to its source. If the obstruction is a result of discharge or suspected wax, the ear should be gently cleaned (preferably by microsuction) and the examination repeated. If there is a mass in the meatus that prevents an adequate view, the examiner must identify its nature.

Difficulty usually arises when there is uncertainty as to whether or not the light is being directed in the correct manner. A good rule with regards to these obstructions is that if an ordinary-sized speculum can touch the object that is obstructing the view then the depth of the drum has not been reached.

The obstruction may be caused by wax. This is readily identifiable by means of its dark-brown, sometimes almost black, coloration, and it can be touched without discomfort to the patient. Furuncles may also obstruct the view of the drum but the extreme sensitiveness in such a case will readily show that acute inflammation is present. A polyp may likewise form an obstruction which is easily reached by the speculum. Polyps are, as a rule, insensitive, and may be moved about by a probe.

Accumulations of debris – such as those encountered in cases of otitis externa – may need to be removed before an adequate view of the drum can be obtained. If anything of this nature obstructs the view, the obstruction should be examined carefully with the aid of a probe. If this is done with sufficient gentleness, no discomfort will be caused to the patient and an accurate diagnosis is more likely.

The greatest difficulties are likely to be encountered in cases where the drum is completely absent. It can be very challenging for the inexperienced examiner to decide whether or not the drum has been reached. The depth of the examined object will sometimes give a clue to its nature, and the remains of the drum will usually be seen when careful examination of the periphery of the meatus is made. Finally, any point of tenderness around the ear must be identified.

Further detailed examination of the ear in the specialist clinic will include microscope assessment. Microsuction can be used at the same time to remove any residual debris which is obscuring the view. An accurate evaluation of chronic middle ear disease cannot be made without the use of the microscope and suction.

EXAMINATION OF THE EUSTACHIAN TUBE

Assessment of eustachian tube function, and thus of middle ear pressure, is an important part of ear examination, especially if a conductive type of hearing loss is present. Some impression can be obtained as described below, and examining the tubal opening by flexible fibreoptic or rigid nasal endoscope is a useful preliminary.

In the Valsalva inflation method the patient keeps the nostrils tightly pinched and attempts to blow out; air enters the eustachian tube. The eardrum is seen to move, and a click is often heard.

The manoeuvre is essential in diving and useful in flying, although many people with normal eustachian tube function cannot master the technique.

Politzer's method consists of applying the olive of a Politzer bag firmly to one nostril and pinching the other side. The patient blows the cheeks and the bag is suddenly pressed to force air up the eustachian tube.

In eustachian catheterisation a suitably curved special metal catheter is passed along the floor of the cocainised nose and when the tip is in the nasopharynx it is slipped laterally into the opening of the eustachian tube. When air is blown in, some idea of Eustachian patency is obtained: a soft clear blowing sound indicates a patent tube; absent sound followed by a blowing one indicates that a blocked tube has been successfully cleared and there will be an immediate hearing improvement. This procedure is now rarely performed.

These tests demonstrate that air can be forced up the eustachian tube, but little else. Manometric studies were formerly regarded as useful, but it is now known that such tests are not helpful in patient selection, nor are they related to the results of tympanoplasty.

Nowadays middle ear pressures can be accurately and quickly diagnosed by tympanometry (p. 15), which has therefore virtually replaced the traditional methods described above for examining the eustachian tube.

EXAMINATION OF HEARING

There are two chief classes of hearing loss, conductive and sensorineural, and the first step is to determine which is present or whether the hearing loss is of a mixed type (Fig. 2.3).

Conductive hearing loss

This results from any interruption to the passage of sound up to and including the stapediovestibular joint.

Sensorineural hearing loss

Terms such as 'nerve deafness' are now outdated. Various components of the sensorineural system

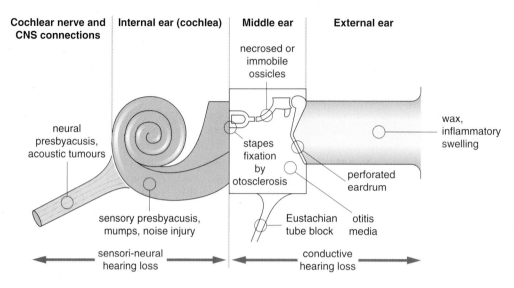

Cochlear nerve and CNS connections | **Internal ear (cochlea)** | **Middle ear** | **External ear**

necrosed or immobile ossicles

neural presbyacusis, acoustic tumours

stapes fixation by otosclerosis

wax, inflammatory swelling

perforated eardrum

sensory presbyacusis, mumps, noise injury

Eustachian tube block   otitis media

sensori-neural hearing loss

conductive hearing loss

Fig. 2.3 Examples of conductive and sensorineural hearing loss and their sites.

are recognised, but special tests are necessary to identify lesions of individual parts. Sensory hearing loss arises when the lesion is in the cochlea; a neural lesion is one that affects the cochlear nerve – the terms cochlear and retrocochlear loss are sometimes used instead. It is important to recognise that lesions may also affect the higher auditory pathways, including the auditory cortex. Furthermore, lesions of the subcortical regions should sometimes be considered. These regions are concerned with the organisation of auditory information, and when deranged may cause language impairment and communication difficulties with no hearing defect as such, or certainly not one which can be recognised by conventional audiometric testing.

Mixed hearing loss

In many instances both types of hearing loss are present. For example, many patients suffering from chronic otitis media or otosclerosis have some degree of cochlear damage as well. In patients with mixed hearing loss, the impairment of the sensorineural reserve clearly places a limit on what the surgeon can do to improve hearing in any reconstructive procedure such as tympanoplasty or stapedectomy. If the sensorineural reserve is seriously affected, any attempt to improve the coexisting conductive hearing loss surgically may accordingly be contraindicated.

Tuning fork tests

Differentiation between the chief types of hearing loss can be made by means of tuning forks. In testing hearing the only useful fork is one of 512 Hz – a 256 Hz fork is not used, although it is neurologically useful for assessing vibration sensation. Although tuning fork tests are valuable in unilateral 'pure' types of loss, the results are difficult to interpret with bilateral or mixed losses.

Rinne's test

This is the most important of the tuning fork tests. Hearing by air conduction is normally better than by bone conduction; air conduction is superior to bone conduction not only in normal patients but also in patients with sensorineural hearing loss. This is a Rinne-positive result. The opposite situation, i.e. hearing better by bone conduction than by air conduction, is a Rinne-negative result, and is found in many patients with conductive hearing loss. If the loss is small, however, the normal Rinne-positive response may still be obtained.

The Rinne test is carried out as follows. A tuning fork is sounded and held beside the ear, the tines parallel to the side of the head and their ends 2 cm from the meatus. The patient is asked to indicate when the sound is no longer heard and the fork is then immediately placed with its base on the mastoid process. If the tuning fork is not heard in this position the patient is Rinne-positive, but if sound is heard again the result is Rinne-negative. The procedure may be reversed or the patient may be asked to compare the intensity of the sound in the two positions and to indicate which is louder. The result is positive if it is louder beside the ear, negative if louder on the mastoid bone.

Warning must be given concerning the 'false-negative' Rinne. In this situation the patient will say that he or she hears the tuning fork better by bone conduction than by air conduction despite having a 'dead' ear (that is, one with a profound or total hearing loss) on the side being examined. This occurs because, when the fork is placed on the mastoid, sound energy is transferred through the bone of the skull to the opposite, functioning cochlea. The patient is unknowingly hearing the sound in the opposite (non-test) ear. The possibility of a false-negative Rinne should always be borne in mind in any patient with an apparently severe unilateral conductive loss, one with apparently bilateral conductive loss or any patient in whom the Weber test (below) is contradictory. A false-negative Rinne is unlikely to be missed if the opposite ear is 'masked' with a Barany noise box.

Weber's test

The tuning fork is sounded and placed in the middle of the patient's head (forehead or vertex). The patient is asked if he or she can hear the sound. If so, where is the sound loudest: in the middle or one or other ear? In a unilateral conductive hearing loss the patient usually points to that ear, or the ear with the greater loss if both have conductive losses.

In sensorineural hearing loss the situation is reversed. The sound is heard more loudly in the ear with the better functioning nerve and cochlea.

Audiometry

The simplest method of assessing hearing is to ascertain how well the patient can hear a conversational voice at varying distances from one ear, the other ear being covered. The usual and more accurate method is some form of audiometry.

The pure-tone audiometer produces a range of pure tones at varying intensity in 5 dB steps. Air conduction thresholds are measured between 250 and 8000 Hz, although the normal human range of hearing extends above this range. Bone conduction thresholds are measured between 250 and 4000 Hz. The latter gives a fairly accurate indication of sensorineural function; they are an important part of any hearing assessment but in particular when surgery for hearing improvement is being considered. The results of pure-tone audiometry are plotted on an audiogram (Fig. 2.4).

The speech audiometer presents speech, in the form of phonetically balanced words, at calibrated volumes. The results are recorded as a percentage of words correctly heard, and repeated for each intensity (Fig. 2.5). This test allows a determination of the patient's ability to discriminate speech. In sensorineural hearing loss the maximum discrimination score is often reduced. In other words, although sound may be perceived at high intensities, words cannot be clearly distinguished. Speech audiometry is valuable in assessing a patient's suitability for surgery and hearing aids.

Tympanometry

Measurement of the compliance and resistance (that is, impedance) of the middle ear mechanism may be used in helping to differentiate between various types of hearing loss. By measuring the degree to which a tone is 'reflected' from the eardrum while varying the pressure in the external ear canal, an indirect measure of middle ear pressure is obtained (Fig. 2.6).

Tympanometry is of great value in assessing children with suspected 'glue ear' (Ch. 4). No special cooperation is required to do the test, apart from the ability to sit still for a few moments while a special probe is inserted into the ear canal. In patients with glue ear a characteristically flat recording is obtained (Fig. 2.6). Tympanometry also allows the stapedius reflex to be examined – the stapedius muscle contracts reflexly when a stimulus of 70 dB above threshold is presented to the ear. If the drum is intact this can be recorded with the tympanometer. If part of the ossicular chain is fixed

Examination and assessment of the ear

(a)

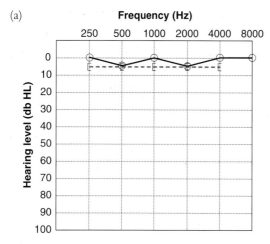

(b)

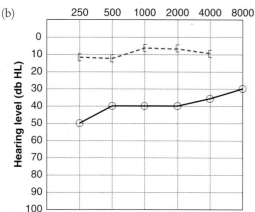

(c)

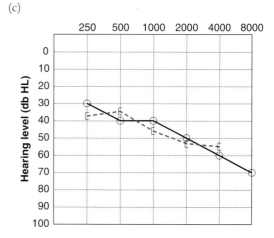

Fig. 2.4 Pure-tone audiograms. (a) Normal hearing in right ear. Frequency (Hertz) is shown on the x axis, hearing level (decibels) on the y axis. Normal hearing is at the top of the graph. The open circles are the standard symbol for right-sided air conduction (the symbol for the left is a cross, X). The square bracket with its side to the right ([) represents right-sided masked bone conduction (the symbol for the left is the reverse,]). (b) Bone conduction is normal but there is an air conduction loss. This is a pure conductive loss. (c) Bone conduction and air conduction are equal and both are below normal. This is a pure sensorineural loss.

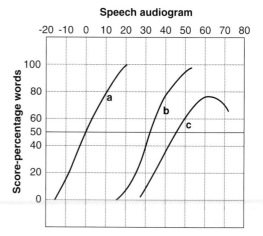

Fig. 2.5 Speech audiogram. The sound level at which words are presented is shown on the x axis, the percentage of words heard correctly on the y axis. (a) Typical curve for patient with normal hearing. (b) Conductive loss: the curve is parallel to curve A but shifted to the right. (c) Sensorineural loss: speech discrimination is never 100%, however loudly words are presented.

(as is the stapes in otosclerosis), no reflex will be demonstrated. In the past the stapedial reflex has also been the basis of tests to differentiate between sensory and neural lesions; these are now rarely performed.

Differential diagnosis

Conventional audiometry is useful for clarifying and documenting the nature and extent of conductive and sensorineural hearing loss. Formerly, special audiometric tests were also used to differentiate the specific site of a sensorineural loss. These are now rarely performed as advances in imaging allow rapid identification of neural pathology. This is discussed further in Chapter 6.

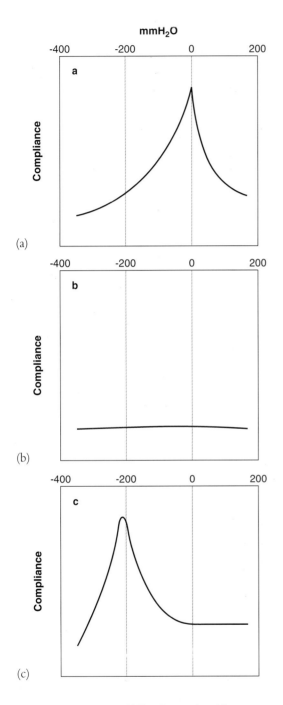

mmH$_2$O

Fig. 2.6 Tympanograms. (a) Type A normal middle ear pressure; (b) Type B flat tracing characteristic of fluid in middle ear or hole in ear drum; (c) Type C negative middle ear pressure as seen with eustachian tube dysfunction.

Tests for non-organic hearing loss

Some patients who appear to have a hearing loss (usually sensorineural) are malingering; they have non-organic hearing loss (NOHL). One of several clinical techniques involving tuning forks and the Barany noise box may be used to try and detect NOHL. The Stenger test, using a pair of tuning forks, is probably the best known – this can also be performed using an audiometer. Some patients with NOHL develop extraordinary skill in misleading clinicians.

Evoked response audiometry

The techniques of evoked response audiometry make possible the objective assessment of hearing. The basic principle is that an auditory stimulus is presented to the ear at regular intervals. Electrodes attached to the skin of the head (surface electrodes) or inserted through the eardrum (transtympanic electrode) are used to record the electrical activity of the cochlea, auditory nerve, brainstem and higher centres. By averaging the recorded responses following many stimuli, the background electrical activity is 'averaged out' to nothing, while any response in synchrony with the stimulus is multiplied.

Electrocochleography records the activity of the cochlea. This has been proposed as a useful test in the diagnosis of patients with Ménière's disease, but the specificity and sensitivity of the test are poor and its diagnostic usefulness unproven.

Brainstem evoked responses are recorded from the auditory nerve and brainstem using surface electrodes. Previously used as a diagnostic tool to detect acoustic neuromas (p. 69), this technique is now rarely used for this purpose. Cortical evoked responses arise from higher centres. They provide a useful objective and frequency-specific measure of thresholds in patients who are difficult to test with behavioural audiometry or are suspected of having NOHL.

EXAMINATION OF VESTIBULAR FUNCTION

A thorough examination of the cranial nerves, cerebellar system, posture and gait must be undertaken in patients with balance problems. A number of specific factors should be evaluated.

Nystagmus

Various types of nystagmus (involuntary, rhythmical, oscillatory eye movements) exist and must be differentiated. Nystagmus arising from vestibular disease usually has two components: a slow labyrinthine component in one direction, and a fast correcting, cerebral or voluntary component in the other. It is nearly always horizontal and is named after the direction of the fast phase. If only seen when the patient's gaze is directed towards the fast phase, it is termed first-degree. In second-degree nystagmus movement is seen even if the patient is looking straight ahead, and in third-degree, when looking away from the direction of the quick component. Vertical nystagmus occurs in central disorders. Acute vestibular failure (from labyrinthitis or a destructive surgical procedure, for example) results in nystagmus with its fast phase away from the affected ear.

Fistula sign

It is especially important to perform the fistula test in patients with vertigo and chronic suppurative otitis media. Pressure is applied to the entrance of the external auditory meatus: this is usually done by pressing the tragus backwards to occlude the canal. A positive result is indicated when vertigo is produced and a deviation of the eyes to the opposite side is observed, with a return when the pressure is withdrawn. There may be occasionally true nystagmus. A positive sign indicates that there is a fistula between the middle and inner ear.

Positional tests

Positional testing should be carried out if the patient's vertiginous symptoms are related to specific movements. The patient sits erect upon a couch in such a position that, when lying down, the head will slightly overhang the end of the couch. The head is turned to one side and the patient is asked to fix his gaze on a point between the examiner's eyes. The examiner holds the patient's head and the patient is then laid down quickly, the head assum-

ing a position just below the horizontal. The patient reports any sensation of vertigo and the examiner notes any nystagmus. The test is repeated with the head turned in the opposite direction. It is important that the examiner bends down to the patient's level while doing the test so that the patient does not move the eyes from the neutral, straight-ahead position.

Characteristic findings are present in patients with benign positional paroxysmal vertigo (Ch. 6).

TESTS OF VESTIBULAR FUNCTION

Tests of vestibular function are useful but it must be appreciated that they do not distinguish between pathology of the labyrinth and of the vestibular nerve. Furthermore, they do not examine the function of the entire labyrinth.

Caloric tests

Caloric testing depends upon the production of convection currents in the semicircular canals by heating or cooling the labyrinth. It can be performed by carefully irrigating the ear with hot or cold water, or insufflating hot or cold air.

The patient lies on a couch with the head raised 30° above the horizontal; this brings the horizontal semicircular canal to the vertical position. In Kobrak's test, 2 ml of cold water are delivered from a syringe on to the posterosuperior segment of the drum under direct vision. The resulting nystagmus is timed and the test repeated on the opposite side. This is a useful, if rather gross, bedside test of vestibular function.

In Hallpike bithermal caloric testing the ears are irrigated in turn with warm (44°C) and cold (30°C) water for 40 seconds. The duration of nystagmus is recorded. The direction of the nystagmus can be recalled from the mnemonic COWS: Cold, Opposite; Warm, Same. The advantage of caloric testing is that both ears can be tested separately. This method is useful for comparing vestibular function in one ear with that in the other (Fig. 2.7).

Electronystagmography

This is a means by which a permanent recording of nystagmus can be made and it is dependent on the

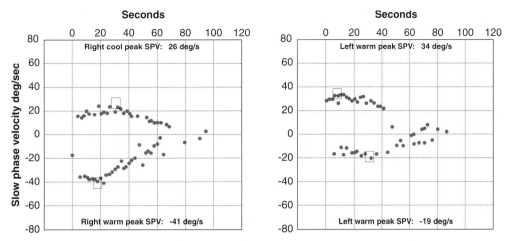

Fig. 2.7 Results of caloric testing plotted by a computerised system. The degree of induced nystagmus (*y* axis) is plotted against time (*x* axis) for the two ears, with both warm and cold stimulation. The degree of canal paresis can be calculated.

presence of a potential difference between the cornea and retina. Electrodes attached around the orbit accurately record eye movements. As well as enabling an exact analysis of speed, amplitude and frequency of eye movement, the test allows detection of nystagmus which may not be visible to the naked eye. Nystagmus of labyrinthine origin can be suppressed by fixation. Electronystagmography (ENG) done in darkness makes detection more likely. Spontaneous nystagmus of central origin is inhibited in darkness. ENG can be used to record nystagmus in response to positional testing, caloric stimulation, etc. Abnormal patterns may be seen when the patient tries to follow a swinging pendulum or when optokinetic nystagmus is being examined. Such abnormalities are important in the diagnosis of lesions of the vestibular nuclei and brainstem.

Rotatory chair tests

A rotating chair can be used to evaluate horizontal semicircular canal function. The patient is seated upright in a special chair with the head tilted 30° down, and several different stimulation paradigms are available: it stimulates both canals simultaneously. The test is usually well tolerated and may be performed on infants and children.

> ➤ **Key points**

- ➤ Adequate examination of the ear is possible only when the entire eardrum can be seen; wax must be removed.
- ➤ Tuning fork tests are useful for distinguishing between types of hearing loss.
- ➤ Pure-tone audiometry provides a good measure of the type and degree of hearing loss.
- ➤ In patients with balance problems a thorough examination of the cranial nerves, cerebellar system, posture and gait must be undertaken.

External ear

3

CONGENITAL ABNORMALITIES

The auricle develops from a series of six tubercles that form around the dorsal margins of the first and second branchial arches. Anomalies of development may be associated with others in the middle or inner ear or congenital malformation of the face and lower jaw.

Preauricular sinuses and cysts

These occur in the region of the crus helicis and are a result of incomplete fusion of the tubercles. They may be complicated by recurrent infection and must then be completely excised.

Accessory auricles

These are the result of anomalous tubercle growth on the branchial arches. They are usually found in the preauricular region but may occur anywhere along a line extending down to the sternoclavicular joint. They may appear to be simple skin tags but frequently contain cartilage.

Bat ear

This is the most common congenital deformity of the pinna. The condition is usually bilateral and may result in children being teased at school. Surgical correction is generally satisfactory. Slightly less common is 'lop' ear, in which the superior part of the pinna appears to be falling forwards; this is somewhat more difficult to correct surgically.

Microtia or anotia

In microtia a more major deformity is present (Fig. 3.1): the pinna may be absent or small and deformed or consist of only a few skin tags. Its position is also frequently abnormal, usually being anterior and low set. Such major abnormalities are always associated with atresia of the external audi-

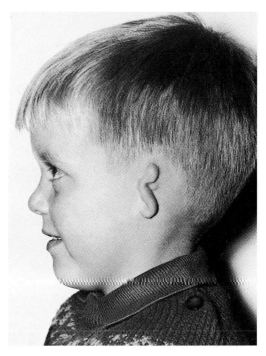

Fig. 3.1 Congenital atresia of the ear. In spite of the severe deformity of the pinna and total bony occlusion of the external meatus, the middle ear and ossicles were relatively normal and the internal ear was entirely normal.

tory canal. It is important to remember, however, that the external ear, the middle ear and the inner ear differ not only in their embryological origins but also in their times of development. This accounts for the wide variation in the types of abnormality, for it is not unusual to see patients with an absent auricle and external auditory canal who are found to have only a moderately severe deformity of the middle ear and its contents, and who have normal inner ears. On the other hand, children may be encountered who have a normal or almost normal external ear and, at the same time, congenital malformation of the middle or inner ear. Abnormalities may be unilateral or bilateral and may be associated with other congenital malformations, such as Treacher Collins syndrome. The deformities may arise from genetic disorders, from a virus, or from toxic drugs acting during early pregnancy. In many cases, however, the cause of the abnormality cannot be determined.

The management of these patients includes assessment and treatment of any hearing impairment as well as management of the cosmetic deformity. If the problem is bilateral and both inner ears are normal, there will be a conductive hearing impairment of the order of 60 dB. Surgical reconstruction of the external meatus and middle ear is complex and not always successful, and long-term hearing improvement is frequently disappointing. The new meatus often has a tendency to be unstable or even to restenose. It is therefore preferable that a bone-conduction hearing aid be prescribed; this may be worn on a hairband. Alternatively, a hearing aid can be anchored directly to the temporal bone by a titanium screw (Ch.7).

Surgical management of the cosmetic deformity is usually delayed until the child is at least of school age. Options include surgical reconstruction using a combination of costal cartilage and skin grafts, or an aural prosthesis, which again can be secured directly into the skull using titanium screws.

ACQUIRED DISORDERS

Injuries to the pinna

Trauma to the pinna may result in a simple laceration or partial or complete avulsion. The only obvious abnormality sometimes is a swelling resulting from the formation of a haematoma – an extravasation of blood between the cartilage and overlying perichondrium. The pinna appears swollen and blue. The outline of the conchal folds is lost and the ear may be slightly tender with a feeling of heat and discomfort. If untreated, the pinna may become distorted and thickened as the haematoma resolves. A 'cauliflower ear' – so often seen in boxers – may result.

Treatment consists of aspiration or drainage of the swelling. If the swelling is liquefied this is most easily done with a syringe and large-bore needle. If a solid or organised clot is present, it should be opened and evacuated under strict aseptic conditions. Whichever method is adopted, a firm pressure dressing is applied in an attempt to discourage more blood from collecting.

After partial or complete avulsion the pinna can sometimes be reattached, otherwise a bone-anchored prosthesis can be fitted.

Infections of the pinna

Perichondritis

Perichondritis is inflammation of the covering of the cartilage, the perichondrium. Infection may produce inflammation in various ways, following infection of a haematoma or other injury, or complicating severe otitis externa. It is an occasional complication of mastoid surgery when cartilage is cut in the presence of gross infection. The pinna is uniformly enlarged and thickened and its surface is red and shiny. There is great pain and frequently considerable constitutional disturbance.

A broad-spectrum antipseudomonal antibiotic is given pending the culture of the infecting organisms. Local treatment consists of the application of soothing dressings such as glycerine and ichthammol. A subperichondrial abscess may be present. If fluctuation is definitely present, the abscess should be incised and drained. Premature incision may result in further spread of infection and more extensive cartilage necrosis.

Skin infections

Skin infections of the pinna are unusual except as a complication of otitis externa.

Impetigo is an infection of the superficial layers of the skin by staphylococci and most commonly occurs in young children. It is frequently secondary to an episode of otorrhoea, and treated with a topical antibiotic. Any causative otorrhoea must be controlled.

Erysipelas is a streptococcal infection that produces raised, red oedematous eruptions with a characteristically sharply defined edge. Blisters are also typical and the condition is usually associated with severe malaise and a high temperature. Treatment with penicillin produces a rapid response.

Dermatitis of the pinna may complicate severe otitis externa. The inflamed skin may become infected by various organisms, and the condition aggravated when the patient becomes sensitised to locally applied eardrops. Treatment is often protracted and difficult because of the severity of the underlying external otitis. Control of this is essential and intensive treatment is usually required. The inflamed skin of the pinna should be cleaned and a topical steroid ointment applied. In particularly difficult cases the help of a dermatologist should be sought. It may be necessary to arrange patch testing to determine if the patient is allergic to one of the components of the local preparations.

Furunculosis occasionally occurs on the pinna. As elsewhere, it is a staphylococcal infection of a hair follicle, generally localised and extremely painful. Deep extension may give rise to perichondritis. The local application of glycerine and ichthammol is helpful. If pus forms, the abscess should be drained.

Herpes

Herpes may occur around the auricle as part of herpes zoster oticus (Ramsay Hunt syndrome; Chapter 8). The vesicles heal spontaneously but a painful neuralgia may precede or follow their eruption.

Tuberculosis

Lupus of the auricle is always accompanied by lesions on the face or mucous membranes. The appearances are those of lupus elsewhere (apple-jelly nodules and scarring), with a tendency to

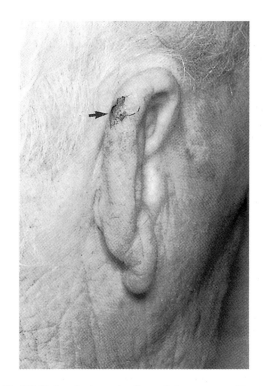

Fig. 3.2 Various benign and malignant lesions occur at this site and in their early stages can appear very similar.

resolution in one part and extension in another. On the ear there is a tendency to ulceration and cartilage destruction.

Tumours of the pinna

Squamous cell and basal cell carcinomas occur on the pinna, often on the edge (Fig. 3.2). Sun exposure with hyperkeratosis is a predisposing factor. Treatment is by excision and/or radiotherapy and should be supervised by a head and neck oncology team.

The external auditory meatus

Wax

Wax in the ear is secreted by glands situated in the skin of the ear – it is nature's provision for the removal of dust and other foreign material from the auditory canal. Excessive wax may sometimes be formed, or wax may be of abnormal consistency, as a result of which it collects in the ear. Wax is normally produced in only a moderate amount and extruded by the movement of chewing and by underlying epithelial migration laterally. It is more commonly found in those with dusty occupations.

Excess wax may cause a variety of symptoms, the chief of which is hearing loss. Pain and irritation in the ear may occur, especially if, on rare occasions, the wax presses on the drum. The sudden onset of hearing loss is explained by the fact that, where only a small space exists between the wax and the meatal wall, a sudden movement or the ingress of fluid and swelling of the wax may occlude the passage.

Treatment consists of removing the wax. This can be achieved by the careful use of a wax curette or by the more usual method of syringing. If wax is unduly hard, preliminary softening with drops may be useful. Sodium bicarbonate, olive oil or a proprietary preparation, which can occasionally irritate the skin, may be used.

Syringing is not always simple and can easily be performed incorrectly. The stream of water is directed upwards and backwards along the posterior wall of the meatus. It is supposed to go *beyond* the obstructing wax, and then wash out the latter as it comes back outwards along the canal. It goes without saying that if there is no space between the wax and the canal wall this will not happen, and a lump of wax can be driven deeper into the canal, causing distress. Equally, a jet directed straight at the drum under too great a pressure may rupture it.

After wax has been removed, careful inspection of the meatus must be made. In practically all cases examination of the drum membrane after syringing will show a degree of injection of the membrane around the lateral process of the malleus and along the handle; this must not be confused with an early otitis media.

Keratosis obturans

In this condition wax accumulates in the deep part of the external meatus, and with continued desquamation of the epithelium a mass is formed. This consists of wax and epithelium which contains cholesterol and exerts pressure on surrounding tissues. By continued enlargement the keratotic mass causes progressive erosion and expansion of the bony meatus and may go on to invade the middle ear. The mass may be fairly silent until an external otitis supervenes and causes severe pain. The ring of granulation tissue that forms superficial to the expanding keratotic mass is almost diagnostic. Removal may be accomplished by careful softening of the mass, but in most cases a general anaesthetic is required. The condition may occur alone or as part of a syndrome with sinusitis and bronchiectasis.

Otitis externa

This is a generalised inflammation involving the skin of the external auditory canal, including the surface of the tympanic membrane. It may be primary, or secondary to a middle ear infection, when the flow of mucopus from the middle ear irritates and infects the external canal skin. Infection is not always present: an eczematous otitis externa may occur in the same way that eczema and seborrhoeic dermatitis occur in other parts of the body. The condition is often painful and an aural discharge may be present.

Certain conditions predispose to otitis externa. Infections are common in hot, humid climates; dust and other irritants lead to irritation and scratching of the ears, an abrasion results and organisms can enter. A tendency to eczema or seborrhoeic dermatitis may exist. Getting the ears wet and then being unable to dry the canals satisfactorily may precipitate external otitis. Sensitisation to the antibiotic content of drops initially used for treatment may prolong inflammation. In unilateral cases, underlying middle ear disease must be excluded. In severe recurrent disease it is wise to exclude diabetes.

A wide variety of organisms may be cultured, including haemolytic streptococcus, *Staphylococcus aureus* and *Pseudomonas* spp.; however, the role of these organisms in the pathogenesis of the condition is not always clear.

In the acute infective condition the diagnosis is simple. The meatus is acutely inflamed, tender and weeping freely, it is extremely painful to handle and nothing can be seen of the interior of the canal without causing the patient pain. No conclusions can be drawn at this stage about the possible causes of the problem, and treatment is directed towards soothing inflamed tissues. In less acute forms there is swelling and redness of the skin of the external auditory canal and the canal may be filled with debris. The ear is tender to touch and the glands in front of or behind the ear may be enlarged. The drum may or may not be visible, but as a rule hearing loss is not marked. This observation is of prime importance because otitis media may be present and be the cause of the maceration and infection of the canal skin. In very minor cases the only sign of disease may be a little crusting and scaling of the epithelium.

In advanced cases, pain is one of the outstanding characteristics and analgesics combined with the local application of heat are helpful. In severe cases a broad-spectrum antibiotic should be given. Local treatment depends on the condition of the canal. If the canal is obstructed by debris, this should be removed under direct vision using the operating microscope. The drum can then be visualised and treatment prescribed and instilled. A variety of drops consisting of antibiotic–steroid combinations, as well as creams and ointment, are available. Caution must be exercised when considering the use of antibiotic-containing drops if a perforation exists – some of the antibiotics are potentially ototoxic and carry a theoretical risk to hearing if they enter the middle ear.

In simple cases, thorough cleaning followed by a short course of antibiotic steroid drops is usually adequate. If there is no suggestion of infection, simple steroid drops are preferred. If the canal is very swollen, a small foam wick can be inserted for a few days. Traditionally, strips of ribbon gauze impregnated with 8% aluminium acetate or ichthammol and glycerine have been used, and these may need to be changed daily. As an alternative, creams or ointments may be instilled into the canal under direct microscopic vision every 4–7 days.

Malignant otitis externa is an extreme form of otitis externa seen in immunocompromised patients (such as elderly diabetic patients). It is caused by *Pseudomonas* spp. Osteomyelitis of the skull base may occur and the condition requires intensive treatment in hospital.

Whatever the origin, external otitis not due to underlying middle ear disease is often bilateral and chronic and the condition is usually demanding for both doctor and patient. Prevention is important. The patient must keep the ears as dry as possible and avoid poking anything into the ear; even simple syringing is probably best avoided. At the earliest sense of itching or discomfort the patient should seek medical attention, and if the canal is occluded by debris or wax this should be removed. A short course of topical steroid, with or without antibiotic as appropriate, should be prescribed. Since allergic reactions to the antibiotics are not uncommon, a patient in whom this is suspected (and the index of suspicion should be high) should be referred to a dermatologist for patch testing.

The otologist occasionally sees patients in whom gross stenosis of the canal has occurred in response to repeated infections, and this can prevent access for treatment. In such cases total excision of the hypertrophic, chronically inflamed skin, together with a meatoplasty, widening of the bony meatus and skin grafting, can be curative.

Furunculosis

This is a hair follicle infection and so can occur only in the skin of the outer part of the meatus. The outstanding symptom is acute pain, which may spread up the side of the head, into the jaw, or down the neck. It may be so severe as to deprive the patient of any hope of rest. There is swelling of the parts around the ear, corresponding to the location of the boil within the meatus. If it is in the anterior wall, the tissue in front of the tragus is swollen; if behind, the oedema may spread over the mastoid process, or above to the temporal region, superficially resembling acute mastoiditis. Tenderness on pressure is marked the tenderness is found more in front of the ear and below than on any other part. The acute pain produced by movement of any part of the cartilaginous meatus is typical of this condition, for any movement of the cartilage naturally puts tension upon the extremely painful tissues lining the ear. Hearing is impaired only when the furuncle is of sufficient size to occlude the external auditory canal completely.

Because of the swelling it is frequently difficult to view the deep meatus. The walls appear to be in apposition, and on attempting to introduce the speculum extreme pain is produced. If examination is carefully pursued it will be seen that the swelling is confined to one or other wall; if the condition has advanced, a discharging point may be seen when the furuncle has burst, and it may be possible to express pus from its opening. The most difficult types of furuncle to diagnose are the deep-seated, early types, in which there is little to be seen on superficial examination. The canal appears to be wide open, the drum membrane may be normal, but if examination is carried out carefully a small swelling or fullness will usually be found in the floor or other aspect of the canal. If probed, there is usually a definite spot of tenderness.

Treatment is with strong analgesia, oral antibiotics (amoxycillin is the usual drug of choice) and the application of a soothing wick, such as one soaked in ichthammol and glycerine.

Otomycosis

Fungal infections are found in the external auditory canal, either as primary disease or complicating otitis externa. The usual organism is *Aspergillus albicans* or *A. niger*. The presence of masses of material like wet paper, upon which mycelia can be seen, is characteristic. The colour of the mass may be white, through brown to black. The condition responds to careful cleaning (preferably by microsuction) and use of a fungicide such as nystatin or clotrimazole. Local treatment must be continued for at least 3 weeks after apparent cure in order to eradicate fungal spores, otherwise recurrence is inevitable. The presence of a fungal infection should always be suspected in otitis externa that appears resistant to treatment. This is especially true if antibiotic–steroid drops have been used as these may precipitate fungal infection.

Foreign bodies

Foreign bodies in the ear are almost invariably confined to children. They may be of vegetable or non-vegetable origin. While syringing may be used to remove the latter, there is always a risk that vegetable material may swell if syringed, so these objects are best removed under direct vision. Some foreign bodies (beads or stones for example) can be removed using small hooks. Crocodile forceps should be avoided in the case of smooth, rounded objects as they may simply push the body further in. In small children it is wise to give them a short general anaesthetic as it is impossible safely to remove a foreign body from a wriggling, struggling child. If the appropriate facilities are not at hand the patient should be referred to a specialist unit.

Exostosis

Exostoses are usually multiple and bilateral, affecting chiefly the anterior and posterior walls. An exostosis is a bony outgrowth from the wall of the external auditory meatus: it may be composed of cancellous or compact bone. The condition is frequently found in swimmers, and the patient may be completely unaware of their existence, or, on the other hand, may come for advice regarding hearing loss, when it may be found that the meatus is completely blocked by new bone. External otitis or impaction of wax may be responsible for the final closure of the meatus.

Treatment can be difficult. A single, pedunculated exostosis is generally straightforward to remove, but removal of multiple exostoses is not to be undertaken lightly, and requires microsurgical procedures. The anterior exostosis, in cases where these are multiple, is usually in contact with the tympanic membrane on its deep surface, so great care is required to avoid damage to this structure. Even more serious is the fact that a severe sensorineural hearing loss may occur if the rotating burr of the drill should momentarily touch the handle of the malleus. When each of the exostoses has been drilled off, any skin flaps that have survived are carefully replaced; alternatively, free grafts may be applied in order to avoid soft tissue stenosis.

An exostosis of the posterior wall must be distinguished from an osteoma arising in the mastoid itself. Management of such an osteoma demands a degree of skill because there is a danger of damage to the facial nerve.

Tumours

Malignant disease of the external auditory canal is much rarer than disease of the pinna itself, but malignant polyps may present which have their origin in the middle ear or the mastoid cavity. They are nearly always the result of prolonged suppuration. Malignancy is to be suspected, especially in older patients in whom there is a fleshy-looking polyp that bleeds easily or if pain seems unusually severe.

Treatment of these patients is always difficult and often disappointing. An extended radical mastoidectomy combined with radiotherapy probably constitutes the best treatment, but extensive or recurrent tumours can sometimes only be controlled by a total petrosectomy.

> ➤ **Key points**
> - ➤ A haematoma of the pinna should be treated to prevent a 'cauliflower ear'.
> - ➤ Allergy to a topical preparation may be responsible for intractable inflammation of the pinna or external canal.
> - ➤ Wax is normal.
> - ➤ Cleaning the ear – by microsuction if necessary – is an important part of the treatment of otitis externa.
> - ➤ Remove foreign bodies in the external canal with great caution.
> - ➤ Be suspicious of crusted, bleeding lesions on the pinna.

Tympanic membrane and middle ear

4

TYMPANIC MEMBRANE

The tympanic membrane may be involved in many conditions affecting the external ear lateral to it, or the middle ear deep to it.

Infections

Otitis externa

The membrane may be involved as part of this condition. It loses its lustre, becomes thickened and sometimes pink. The surface desquamates, the epithelium coming off in flakes and giving the drum a rough, whitish appearance. Oedema can be so marked as to obscure the landmarks – sometimes a localised area of myringitis occurs which can become chronic and cause suspicion of an adjacent area of osteitis. When the infection of the meatus is brought under control, the drum will also improve; after repeated or prolonged attacks, however, the drum may be permanently thickened.

Bullous myringitis

This is often seen during influenza epidemics and has been assumed to be caused by a virus infection; this remains unproven. Serious intracranial complications may occasionally ensue. Haemorrhagic bullae are found on the drum and may spread to the wall of the meatus, usually on the posterosuperior aspect. These appear as dark bluish or red swellings which may be small, or large enough to obscure the drum completely. At first the hearing may be unaffected and the chief complaint is of acute pain. The pain is extremely severe, preventing sleep or work and may completely incapacitate the patient. When the bullae burst, the pain ceases and there is bleeding from the ear. Later, as the bullae heal, any remaining clot turns into blackish crusts. Acute otitis media – or more rarely viral labyrinthitis or meningoencephalitis – may occur. Treatment consists of analgesia and keeping the ear dry.

Herpes

The membrane is affected in herpes zoster oticus (q.v.).

Trauma

Perforations may be caused by foreign bodies of various kinds (hairpins or other instruments) being pushed through the drum from the external meatus: they may do this when misguided attempts are being made to remove them. Matches are a known cause of injury, which may occur if a patient receives a jog in the elbow while scratching the ear with a match. A blow on the ear or compression of

29

Tympanic membrane and middle ear

air in the external meatus may be sufficient to rupture the drum. A gunshot blast may cause sufficient air displacement to rupture the drum, either inwards by direct blast or outwards by blast suction. In the latter case the edges of the rupture are seen to be everted. A tear in the eardrum can occur with a fracture of the petrous bone which runs through the middle ear and deep meatus. Long after the drum has healed, a displaced fracture line remains visible.

Treatment

If facilities permit there is much to be said in favour of examining with an operating microscope any ear that has received a penetrating injury. This can generally be done in the outpatient clinic. Wax or debris in the ear canal can be removed and the drum visualised. Treatment is usually straightforward, and in general the less that is done the better. A sterile dressing should be applied to the entrance of the external canal. If the wound is 'clean', no medication is necessary. If infection has been introduced into the middle ear, appropriate antibiotic–steroid eardrops should be prescribed. On no account should the ear be syringed. The drum usually heals spontaneously, but if not it can be repaired later. The ossicular chain can be reconstructed if this too has been damaged.

Urgent exploration of the ear by formal tympanotomy is essential firstly, if there is any evidence of injury to the facial nerve; and secondly if giddiness, nystagmus or sensorineural hearing loss has been caused by the injury. In such patients subluxation of the stapes footplate is probable – failure to repair the oval window will almost certainly result in a dead ear with permanent hearing loss.

Retraction pockets and atelectasis

The normal drum is tense, apart from the pars flaccida superiorly, and it is covered by a thin layer of desquamated epithelial cells. These two features result, firstly, from the presence of the middle elastic layer in the pars tensa and, secondly, from the normal migration of the epithelial layer from the drum along the meatal wall to the exterior. One or both of these features may be disturbed by mechanisms that are not fully understood. Damage to the middle layer of the drum may result from middle ear infections – this is especially seen in otitis media with effusion. Continuing impairment of middle ear aeration due to inadequate eustachian tube function may produce atelectasis – a process in which part of the drum becomes thin and retracts medially into the middle ear space. This process may be diffuse but occurs most readily in the posterosuperior segment of the drum. Initially, retraction produces a shallow depression in the drum but this can develop into a deeper pocket (Fig. 4.1). As long as these pockets remain small and there is no retention within them of the epithelial debris which their lining produces, it may be safe to keep them under observation. Severe atelectasis can sometimes be reversed if middle ear pressure is artificially maintained by a long-term ventilating grommet. Insertion of such a grommet may be justified, even if 'glue' is no longer present in the middle ear cleft. In many children, it appears that the middle layer of the eardrum has substantial powers of recovery and regeneration. Unless adhesions have already formed between the medial surface of the drum and the middle ear contents, the pars tensa may again become tense and regain its normal appearance and position.

In deep retraction pockets, on the other hand, adhesions may prevent successful eversion of the pockets, the self-cleaning mechanism may fail and there will be an accumulation of epithelial debris (Fig. 4.1). This accumulated debris must be recognised and removed to encourage the self-cleaning mechanism to recover. Failure to do so will result in the development of cholesteatoma (q.v.). It is now thought that the majority of cholesteatomas begin in this way.

Retraction pockets and cholesteatoma are discussed further below in the context of chronic suppurative otitis media (this may be of various types). With the newer classification system, based on pathological considerations, two forms of 'squamous epithelial chronic otitis media' are recognised: an active type, synonymous with cholesteatoma, and an inactive type, which includes retraction pockets.

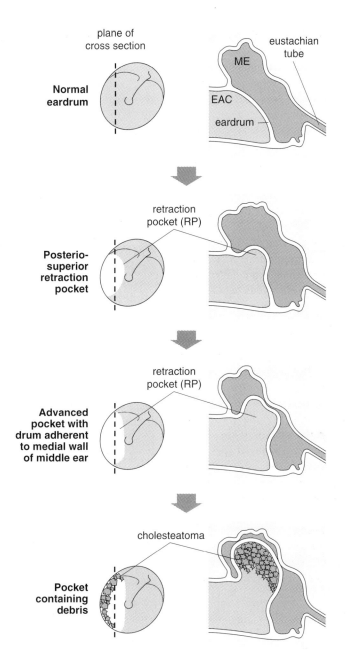

Fig. 4.1 Otoscopic view of right tympanic membrane (left) and sagittal section along dotted line (right). ME: middle ear, EAC: external auditory canal.

Perforations

Perforations of the tympanic membrane may arise in several ways: from trauma, as described above; as a consequence of retraction pocket formation (see above); or following a middle ear infection when pus under pressure bursts the eardrum.

It is not always clear from the history how a perforation arose or, more importantly, whether or not there is any sinister or serious middle ear or mastoid pathology underlying it. A clue may be obtained from the *type* of perforation. Perforations are usually single (multiple perforations are supposed to suggest tuberculosis) and are described as being central, marginal or attic.

Central perforation

In this type of perforation a rim of normal drum is visible all round the perforation and the fibrous annulus remains intact (Fig. 4.2). The perforation may be large or small. Frequently the handle of the malleus may be seen projecting into the perforation, which is described as anterior, inferior or posterior according to its position – a kidney-shaped ('reniform') perforation is larger. The defect is sometimes so great as to merit the term 'subtotal' perforation. These types of perforation are usually seen in chronic suppurative otitis media of the tubotympanic type, whether active or quiescent: perforations associated with acute otitis media are always central.

Marginal perforations

These are perforations at the margin of the drum, in which the fibrous annulus is involved (Fig. 4.3). This means that bony disease is present; such perforations are inevitably associated with osteitis, and often with granulations and cholesteatoma formation. The perforation is frequently in reality the mouth of a cholesteatoma or a retraction pocket extending into the middle ear or mastoid: these may be small or large – the size being impossible to assess on examining the drum. Cholesteatoma

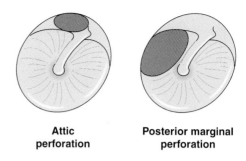

Attic perforation   **Posterior marginal perforation**

Fig. 4.3 'Unsafe' type, tympanic membrane perforations.

debris may be recognised by its white, wax-like appearance and its foul smell. Marginal perforations are usually seen posteriorly. In some cases destruction of the drum margin may allow squamous epithelium to grow from the meatus into the middle ear cavity.

Attic perforations

Attic perforations are situated in the pars flaccida (Fig. 4.3), and are almost invariably associated with an invading cholesteatoma, the perforation representing the mouth of the cholesteatoma sac. Symptoms can be minimal, so that the presence of the disease lies unsuspected – there may sometimes be a slight hearing loss or a little intermittent discharge. An attic perforation should be looked for just above the lateral process of the malleus: it may be pinhole in size, but it can involve the entire pars flaccida, and sometimes also the adjacent bony outer attic wall. The perforation may be obscured by a small brown crust resembling a piece of wax. If on examination the only wax to be seen in the ear is located in the roof and near the drum, its removal will often reveal an attic defect. Although small, such a defect may be associated with a large cholesteatoma. Similar to marginal perforations, these attic defects probably originate from the part of the drum concerned collapsing or being dragged inwards. Although infection and discharge may be minimal, both types of perforation are always associated with chronic, progressive, destructive middle ear disease and osteitis. Occasionally, a patient may be seen with either meningitis or a temporal lobe abscess as the first sign of trouble.

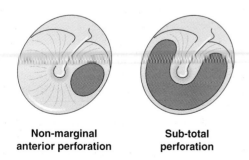

Non-marginal anterior perforation   **Sub-total perforation**

Fig. 4.2 'Safe' type, tympanic membrane perforations.

Examining perforations

If an ear discharges and there are no signs of external otitis, there must be a perforation and the examiner should be able to find it. More erroneous diagnoses are made because the ear has not been adequately cleaned than for any other reason. The drum must therefore be carefully cleaned before a diagnosis can be made.

At the initial examination, the amount of discharge and the severity of the infection very often make accurate examination impossible. In such patients aural toilet, followed by the use of antibiotic–steroid drops, helps suppress infection so that on re-examination a more exact assessment is possible. Indeed in the case of a central perforation the ear may be completely clean and dry when the patient next attends.

A perforation can sometimes be difficult to localise, especially if it lies in the anterior segment, obscured by the anterior canal wall. In such instances it may be helpful if the patient inflates the ear by the Valsalva method (p.13) – this may be sufficient to cause secretions to exude from the perforation. Alternatively, an aspirating speculum may be used to draw the contents of the middle ear through the perforation.

Once the perforation has been found, certain details must be clarified. This is sometimes possible with an otoscope alone but if the patient is being assessed in hospital (and especially if surgery is contemplated) the operating microscope must be used.

First it must be decided whether the perforation is central, marginal or attic. Its size and exact site must be recorded, as well as the condition of the drum remnant, the condition of the middle ear mucosa and the state of the ossicles, which may be visible through the defect. In the case of marginal or attic perforations the presence of any obvious cholesteatoma outside or cholesteatoma will be noted, together with any areas of bony defect.

It must be emphasised again that marginal and attic perforations are characteristic of a progressive disease associated with bone destruction that is potentially dangerous and which nearly always demands surgical treatment, not only to render the ear safe but also to prevent continuing destruction of hearing.

EUSTACHIAN TUBE DYSFUNCTION

The eustachian tube plays an important part in the physiology of the middle ear, and is frequently of primary importance in the cause of diseases of the ear.

Acute obstruction

The role of eustachian tube obstruction in otitis media with effusion in childhood is discussed elsewhere. In adults, acute tubal obstruction often occurs with a cold – even if no middle ear effusion develops, a conductive-type hearing loss may result and the ear can be painful. If temporarily superimposed on another type of hearing loss (especially sensorineural loss in the elderly), a moderate degree of hearing loss can become severe. Tubal dysfunction may also occur when greater than normal demands are placed on the middle ear ventilating mechanism. Examples include those changes associated with flying and diving (p. 45).

Treatment of tubal dysfunction consists of treating the cause (for example, a cold). If this does not lead to resolution, topical nasal decongestants may be used. The middle ear may also be reventilated by the Valsalva method of autoinflation, by using the Politzer bag or by eustachian tube catheterisation.

Chronic dysfunction

Chronic eustachian tube problems in adults usually result in serous otitis (otitis media with effusion – q.v.). This may follow an upper respiratory tract infection or be associated with allergy. Occasionally, a lesion in the nasopharynx, such as a carcinoma or lymphoma, may present with a unilateral chronic middle ear effusion. The management of this disorder in adults should therefore include a thorough examination of the nose and paranasal sinuses; blind biopsies of the nasopharynx are advocated in areas in which nasopharyngeal carcinoma is endemic. Grommet insertion is rarely required in adults but, if it is necessary, it can be performed under local anaesthesia. A tendency to chronic eustachian tube problems only shows itself when the patient is subjected to pressure change, such as when flying.

A specific problem of eustachian tube origin is sometimes seen in adult patients who have had a radical mastoidectomy. This procedure was much more common before modern tympanoplasty procedures were introduced. Such patients have often had a discharging ear for many years, and this occurs because the lateral end of the eustachian tube is in direct continuity with the mastoid cavity. A dry, trouble-free ear can be obtained by placing a graft across the exposed mucosa of the middle ear and eustachian tube opening.

ACUTE OTITIS MEDIA

Acute otitis media is an acute inflammation of the lining of the middle ear cleft. It is extremely common in children but can occur at any age – there is nearly always a preceding upper respiratory infection. The speed at which the disease progresses is variable: it is sometimes quite slow; sometimes fulminating, with perforation of the eardrum within a few hours. Nowadays in the UK, with easy access to medical treatment, the disease is much modified and perforation of the eardrum is relatively unusual. The condition includes all grades of infection, from the lowest degree of inflammation up to the formation of frank pus, with all the accompanying changes in the lining membrane. The reader is reminded that in these cases the whole middle ear cleft must be considered as one. The membranous lining in the middle ear is continuous with that which passes through the aditus into the mastoid antrum and the mastoid cells. In the nose – when the mucous lining of the nasal cavity is infected – the lining of the nasal sinuses, being in continuity with that of the nose, shares in the inflammatory reactions. In most cases of middle ear infection, there is also some reaction in the mastoid antrum and cells. The inflammation may stop short at the aditus or in the mastoid antrum: it is however essential in all cases to look upon the inflammation of the various parts as one disease, and not as a disease that only involves the middle ear and may then afterwards involve other parts or structures.

Sources of infection

The eustachian tube is the chief route by which infection reaches the middle ear – the cause of infection in such cases is nasopharyngeal disease. The infection may occasionally be diffuse, as in a coryza, or the causative infection may be in the nose or sinuses. In all of these conditions an ascending infection of the eustachian tube occurs. In the earlier stages the lower end of the tube is involved, but as the salpingitis spreads further the tube becomes blocked and the air within the middle ear is absorbed and replaced by exudate, which may later become purulent.

Although extension along the eustachian tube is nearly always an extension of inflammation in the lining membrane, otitis media may occasionally result from infected secretions being forced up the tube by pressure changes associated with excessive nose blowing, diving, underwater swimming or flying.

Infection may also enter the middle ear from the external auditory meatus if there is a pre-existing perforation of the drum. It is not unusual to see patients who have had a dry perforation for a long period of time reinfecting their ears by swimming. Very occasionally infection may enter from the external meatus if the drum has been ruptured by trauma.

The great frequency of otitis media in children calls for special comment. It is common in children because upper respiratory infections are widespread, especially those affecting the nose and nasopharynx, and in turn these are common because children have not acquired the resistance that adults enjoy. The role of adenoid hypertrophy and infection is still debated. Various immunodeficiency syndromes (including gammaglobulin deficiency) constitute a rare but important cause of recurring respiratory and ear infection in some children, and may be familial.

Microbiology The most common organism is *Streptococcus pneumoniae*, followed by *Haemophilus influenzae* and *Moraxella (Branhamella) catarrhalis*. Viruses probably play an indirect role in the aetiology of acute otitis media.

Symptoms

Pain is the most prominent symptom. In most cases the presence or absence of pain appears to depend to a large extent on the speed of the accumulation of fluid – just as in other parts of the body, the rapid production of tension is responsible for pain. In the middle ear the degree of tension of the drum and the production of that tension in a short space of time causes the acute pain which is so frequently experienced in otitis media. In these cases there is also an added source of irritation from the inflammation in the drum structure or in the formation of bullae, which may form the first stage of infection. The pain is usually described as being of a sharp, lancinate character located in the ear itself, and does not as a rule seem to radiate in the early stages.

Hearing loss is also a constant symptom in cases in which fluid has accumulated in the middle ear. However, in the earliest stages of middle ear inflammation hearing loss may be almost absent. This is the stage of inflammation without any outpouring of secretions. When fluid begins to accumulate, hearing becomes impaired; with further accumulation the normal movement of the ossicles, their ligaments and the membranes covering the ligaments is prevented, and hearing steadily deteriorates – this is one of the most reliable guides in estimating the progress of acute otitis media. A whisper can normally be heard at a distance of 8 metres: moderate impairment of hearing is present when the distance is reduced to about 2 metres; great impairment when a whisper can only just be heard; and severe impairment when a conversational voice is audible at only a metre or two. The hearing loss is of conductive type.

Discharge is the other cardinal symptom, although it occurs only in the most severe cases. Discharge indicates that necrosis of the drum, with consequent perforation, has occurred. The appearance of discharge is usually associated with substantial lessening of pain. This is an indication of the decrease in tension in the drum membrane. The purulent discharge may initially be bloodstained, but later becomes mucopurulent.

Other symptoms may include tinnitus and voice resonance. Giddiness and sickness occasionally occur from irritation of the inner ear. There is always some general disturbance, shown by a rise in temperature and pulse rate, and malaise.

Signs

The diagnosis of acute otitis media rests largely upon the appearance of the drum membrane and will be by inference only if the eardrum cannot be seen properly. The earliest appearance of infection will be found around the malleus, and consists of inflammation of the vessels around the lateral process and the handle. The inflammation spreads until it involves the whole drum, which loses its lustre, changing from grey to greyish pink, and from pink to bright red. The outline of the drum itself is gradually lost, and when the fluid at first accumulates the drum bulges in its posterior aspect. The swelling gradually spreads until it involves the anterior portion of the drum, and finally a condition is found in which the drum appears as a doubled roll, the dimple in the centre representing the point of attachment of the handle of the malleus. By this time the colour may be dark red, and all the landmarks will have vanished. If a drum is examined when it is on the point of bursting, a yellow nipple at the point of a projecting red bulge indicates the part of the drum that is in process of sloughing.

After perforation the diagnosis is usually simplified. The meatus is full of discharge and if this is mopped away it may be seen to be coming from the perforation, although it is not always easy to locate the exact site. There is pulsation of discharge and this is synchronous with the pulse; pulsation is always an indication that an acute process is present and is best detected by watching a light reflex. Hearing is still impaired, but probably showing signs of improvement. Increasing hearing loss at this time may however be an indication that the infection is not settling or that complications are developing. Constitutional disturbance and pyrexia usually improve with perforation, but failure to do so may be a warning of impending complications.

Tuning fork tests are a valuable guide to the presence or absence of middle ear disease. For the purpose of carrying out these tests, it must be assumed that the external meatus is to a great extent clear of obstruction. It is useless to lay any stress on tuning fork tests in cases in which the external meatus is obstructed by furunculosis or wax, but when the drum can be seen they are a valuable aid in deciding upon the presence or absence of disease.

As already observed, the lining of the middle ear is continuous with that of the mastoid antrum and the mastoid cells. Inflammation inside these cells may give rise to tenderness over the bone of the mastoid process, and the more acute the infection in the ear the more probable is tenderness in the bone behind the ear. This is due to the simultaneous inflammatory reaction inside the mastoid antrum and cells.

If recovery takes place and pus or serum is released from the middle ear then, as a rule, the tenderness behind the ear subsides. If not, and if the inflammation of the ear becomes manifestly purulent, the infection within the bone becomes more advanced and passes into the stage called 'mastoiditis'. This will be gone into more fully when we come to deal with complications of middle ear disease.

Otitis media in children

Otitis media is extremely common in infants and young children but diagnosis can be difficult because the patient is unable to articulate. In infants there is often remarkably little to draw attention to the ear: the baby is simply unwell and has a temperature. Accordingly, any infant with an undiagnosed illness or pyrexia must have the ears examined. Restlessness, crying or screaming (at night-time in particular), putting up the hand to the head or rolling the head on the pillow are all signs which should suggest examination; it may be difficult to estimate hearing, and tuning fork tests are of little use until the child is of an age to participate. In some cases, discharge from the ear will solve the problem and relieve pain if the condition has not been identified and treated. The appearance of discharge is in some cases the first sign of the disease.

Treatment

In treating otitis media, the chief aim is the preservation of normal hearing. With antibiotic treatment the danger to life is so reduced that the whole attention may be given to the problem of restoring and safeguarding function. It cannot be too strongly emphasised that mere recovery from acute symptoms is not sufficient. Misuse of antibiotics may give apparently good immediate results, only to cause future loss of hearing. How far treatment has proved successful is gauged by the degree to which the eardrum, tuning fork tests and hearing have returned to normal.

General treatment consists of confining the patient to bed in a warm but adequately ventilated room. Pain relief is important and can be achieved by the use of local heat in the form of warm olive oil eardrops and a hot water bottle, aided by analgesics.

Re-establishment of eustachian tube function is important. Nasal drops and inhalations given 4-hourly are often prescribed, as are oral decongestants and mucolytics. There is, however, no scientific evidence that they influence or expedite resolution of infection.

Antibiotic chemotherapy In the UK it is customary to give an antibiotic almost routinely to children with acute otitis media. Nevertheless, arguments against the routine prescription of antibiotics have been put forward because of the low frequency of serious complications in the UK, together with the fact that spontaneous resolution occurs in about 85% of patients even without treatment, and because of the incidence of side-effects (especially diarrhoea) in up to 25% of children. In some parts of Europe, antibiotics are rarely prescribed; in the USA, their use is almost mandatory.

The arguments advanced to support treatment or non-treatment in developed countries are unlikely to apply in parts of the world where the incidence of serious complications for example acute mastoiditis is higher.

The choice of chemotherapy depends upon the penetration of the drug into the middle ear space, the suspected organism responsible for the infection, and absence of undesirable side-effects.

On the basis of good penetration of the middle ear and likely sensitivity of the organism responsible, amoxycillin constitutes the first choice. In patients sensitive to penicillin, erythromycin or cefixime may be used. If there is a high incidence of beta-lactamase-producing organisms in the population being treated, an alternative treatment is an amoxycillin-clavulanic acid combination. When in doubt, assistance should be sought from a local microbiologist.

If the ear is discharging, a swab should be taken for bacteriological studies of sensitivity, and, if there has been no response to the first choice of chemotherapy, treatment may be altered depending upon the bacteriological report.

Myringotomy In those patients in whom there is excessive pain, in whom the drum remains obviously full and bulging, or in whom the drum remains abnormal or hearing impaired in spite of the disappearance of acute symptoms, then discharge by myringotomy is sometimes advocated. A swab will be taken for bacteriological study and continuing chemotherapy will depend upon the sensitivity ascertained. In some parts of the world, myringotomy plays a major role in the initial management of acute otitis media.

It has been argued that a myringotomy results in a much more satisfactory scar than one occurring after spontaneous perforation, and the probability of good hearing after the operation is very much greater.

Technique of myringotomy Myringotomy for severe acute otitis media is a rare operation in the UK because of the easy access to primary medical care.

When the operation is necessary a good light is essential and an operating microscope preferred. The knife used is of a special design and it is essential that the handle should be angled to give a clear view of the point during the procedure. The incision is semilunar in shape and should commence posterosuperiorly and finish anteroinferiorly. The point of the knife should be passed through the drum only far enough to cut the drum itself; if it is passed far through the membrane there is danger of injury to the structures of the middle ear. In most cases pus appears immediately after the incision. A specimen should be taken for bacteriological purposes, and a strip of ribbon gauze can be inserted to absorb any blood or pus, helping to drain the middle ear by capillary attraction. The wick can be removed within a few hours.

Although it sounds simple to incise the eardrum at the proper place, the beginner must be warned that the incision should be further forward on the bulge of the drum than would appear to be correct. The chief fault in carrying out this operation is to make the cut too far posteriorly; when the drum collapses the incision lies so close to the posterior wall that drainage is seriously impeded. It should be noted that myringotomy consists of making a full-length incision; in paracentesis, by contrast, only a small stab is made. This is often done for diagnostic purposes, or for aspiration of watery fluid in serous otitis.

Following myringotomy an immediate drop in temperature and improvement of general condition are to be expected. The discharge, passing gradually from a purulent condition to a serous one, should clear up in a few days. Before passing a patient as recovered, careful examination of the hearing must be made. It is re-emphasised that recovery is only complete when hearing is back to normal.

Treatment after myringotomy or perforation The object of treatment is primarily adequate drainage, and the drying up of discharge. Pain does not enter into consideration in those cases in which myringotomy or perforation has occurred. Should pain be present at this stage in the disease, treatment does not consist of soothing the pain, but of treating the cause, for subsequent pain, when adequate drainage has been established, is a symptom that indicates extension of disease and must be looked upon as a danger sign. In certain cases, however, a slight recurrence of pain may occur after the perforation. In these cases the perforation has been inadequate to release the whole of the purulent contents of the middle ear, the perforation tends to close, and may be sealed off completely by oedema. It may be necessary to enlarge the opening in the drum to drain the pus. Premature closure by healing of the perforation may also occur and necessitate another myringotomy.

The perforation or opening in the drum may become obstructed if the discharge in the external meatus is allowed to collect. In these circumstances drainage is inadequate and movement of the secretion in the various parts of the ear is prevented. The discharge should therefore be removed. This may be done by one of two methods – dry or wet. In the dry method the canal is cleansed by mopping: this is done by inserting a small wick of cotton wool deep into the external meatus, where it is allowed to remain for a couple of minutes and then replaced. This is repeated until no more mucopus comes out on the cotton wool. Most parents can carry out this treatment if shown how, and if necessary can do it several times daily.

The wet treatment consists of the instillation of hydrogen peroxide drops. These are allowed to remain in the ear for between half a minute and a minute in order to loosen the accumulated discharge, which is then gently syringed out with warm boric lotion and the ear mopped dry. This treatment is carried out daily or, if the discharge is very copious or thick, twice daily.

In the normal process of resolution the discharge gradually becomes thicker and more mucoid, then slowly assumes a more serous appearance and finally dries up. Normally, the condition may pass through these stages in the course of a week or so but it can take 2–3 weeks. On the other hand, it may enter a subacute stage.

The longer the discharge continues, the greater the danger of some permanent damage. Antibiotic–steroid drops may be useful in those patients in whom some residual moisture remains obstinately present. They should be used several times a day after first getting the ear as clean as possible using a wick of cotton wool as described above, and an attempt should be made to drive the drops into the middle ear by pressure on the tragus (see comments on p. 61). Alternatively, boric and iodine powder (0.75% iodine in boric acid powder) may be insufflated; only sufficient to produce a light dusting is necessary.

If the discharge from the ear continues, a search should be made for the condition responsible for its chronicity. This could be found to be nasopharyngeal disease, which in children may be caused by adenoids. Sinusitis is also sometimes responsible, and an inadequate nasal airway with poor aeration of the postnasal space may be found to be at the root of the trouble. These conditions may need to be corrected before recovery can take place.

It is also important to exclude the possibility of a masked mastoiditis, especially if chemotherapy has been given in inadequate dosage or the organisms are only partially sensitive (p.51).

RECURRENT ACUTE OTITIS MEDIA

In children who suffer from recurrent acute otitis, an underlying immunodeficiency or similar systemic problem must be excluded. Any focus of infection in the upper respiratory tract should be similarly eradicated. Two main treatment options are available as alternatives to repeated courses of antibiotics: long-term low dose prophylactic antibiotics, or grommet insertion. A 3-month course of trimethoprim, especially over the winter months, can be very effective. The grommet is effective presumably because ventilation of the middle ear cleft is encouraged, and negative pressures which might otherwise initiate fluid transudation are prevented.

CHRONIC OTITIS MEDIA

Chronic otitis media occurs in various forms: it may be confined to the middle ear mucosa or it may destroy bone. It can be caused by the failure of an acute infection to resolve completely, or sometimes appear to be chronic from first presentation. As with acute otitis media, the entire middle ear cleft and mastoid must be regarded as one unit.

Chronic otitis media can be broadly classified as:

- non-suppurative: secretory otitis media or otitis media with effusion
- suppurative
- tuberculous.

Otitis media with effusion (OME; glue ear)

This describes an accumulation of fluid in the middle ear, occurring in the absence of acute inflammation. It may vary from a thin serous fluid to thick viscid material; hence the term 'glue ear' which is often used clinically – it is also known as secretory otitis media. This is a very common disorder and undoubtedly the most frequent cause of acquired hearing loss in childhood. It is usually bilateral but may be unilateral, and it is often intermittent. The cause is uncertain although chronic low grade infection, poor eustachian tube function and adenoidal infection or hypertrophy have all been implicated.

The most important symptom is impaired hearing but its onset is often insidious and presentation depends on a child's age. In children under 3 years old there may be delayed speech and language development. Older children may be accused of being inattentive and uncooperative. The problem is often first noticed by a schoolteacher or visiting relative, but many cases are only discovered during routine audiometric screening. Children with otitis media with effusion may present with recurrent acute otitis media and the hearing impairment may be relatively asymptomatic.

On examination, the drum may appear fairly normal, even when a magnifying speculum is used. Typically, however, it is dull and may have a yellow tint; fine blood vessels are often seen coursing inwards from the drum margin (Fig. 4.4). The most important and obvious signs are the lack of mobility of the drum when using the pneumatic speculum and the discovery of a negative Rinne test. When these two clinical signs are present the child in most cases has glue ear. In chronic cases, the drum often becomes thinned, atrophic and collapsed.

In otitis media with effusion, tympanometry, which requires no cooperation from the child, is helpful. A type B (flat) trace is diagnostic. Age-appropriate audiometry will usually confirm a hearing loss of the order of 30–50 dB.

Medical treatment, consisting of decongestant therapy, mucolytics and antihistamines, is often tried but seldom successful; long-term low dose antibiotics may, however, be beneficial in up to 50% of cases. Repeated autoinflation may help in older children but this is difficult for the younger child to master. Surgical treatment by grommet insertion is 100% successful in correcting the hearing impairment. It should not be undertaken for asymptomatic glue ear as most children will grow out of the problem by the age of 5 or 6 years, with no sequelae for the tympanic membrane or middle ear. The operation, which is performed under general anaesthesia, consists of an anterior, inferior myringotomy, aspiration of the thick mucoid material and the insertion of a small plastic tube or grommet (Fig. 4.5). The tube provides for adequate ventilation of the middle ear space and is essentially a bypass system for the eustachian tube; it is not a drainage tube. There is little one can do surgically to improve eustachian tube function, although if the adenoids are very large or infected they should be removed, and it

(a)

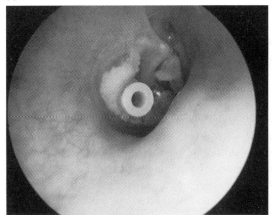

(b)

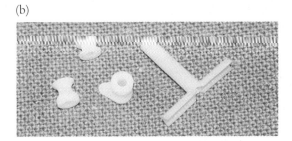

Fig. 4.5 (a) Grommet in situ; (b) various types of ventilating tube ('grommet').

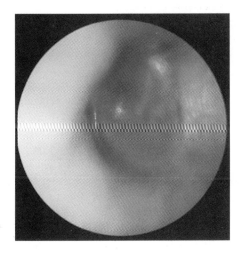

Fig. 4.4 Otitis media with effusion (left ear).

also seems reasonable to treat any chronic inflammation or infection in the nose or paranasal sinuses. As long as the grommet remains in position, the hearing will be normal. After several months, however, the grommet is slowly extruded, and if the eustachian tube function has not yet become normal a recurrence of the effusion may occur in 10–20% of children. If it recurs, again it should only be treated if it is symptomatic.

Some children have a predisposition to poor eustachian tube function; for example, those with a cleft palate or a craniofacial malformation. These patients often require grommet insertion on a number of occasions and the use of a long-term grommet such as a T-tube should be considered in their management. Rarely, a chronic perforation may persist in the tympanic membrane after extrusion of a grommet; this is more common if T-tubes have been used.

Chronic suppurative otitis media

The classification of chronic suppurative otitis media is shown in Box 4.1. The old system of classification has been alluded to above when describing and discussing tympanic membrane perforations.

Mucosal chronic otitis media

When a permanent perforation is left as a result of acute otitis media, this is usually of the 'tubotympanic' or 'safe' variety as there is unlikely to be any sinister underlying middle ear or mastoid problem. If the ear is dry and the middle ear mucosa remains uninflamed and uninfected, the patient has *inactive* mucosal chronic otitis media. If the mucosa becomes inflamed or infected, the disease has become active and the patient has *active* mucosal chronic otitis media.

Active mucosal chronic otitis media Not infrequently this type of middle ear suppuration is accompanied by disease in the nose, sinuses and pharynx. The patient has a discharge, which may be mucoid or mucopurulent. This may be constant or intermittent, reappearing with the onset of upper respiratory infection or the accidental entry of

---

■ Box 4.1

Classification of chronic suppurative otitis media

■ Old system based on *anatomical* considerations	Tubotympanic disease = 'safe' disease; perforation is central and non-marginal
	Atticoantral disease = 'unsafe' disease; perforation is marginal or in attic: cholesteatoma
■ New system based on *pathological* considerations	Healed otitis media
	Inactive mucosal chronic otitis media
	Active mucosal chronic otitis media
	Active squamous epithelial chronic otitis media: cholesteatoma
	Inactive squamous epithelial chronic otitis media: retraction pocket

---

water into the ear. After repeated exacerbations the ossicular chain will usually be eroded, at least in part, and this may be visible through the perforation. In acute exacerbations the middle ear mucosa may be swollen and oedematous and may on occasion produce polyps. There is usually, but not always, a conductive hearing loss. There is no evidence of cholesteatoma.

Medical treatment is directed at drying up the discharge. In addition to local treatment this may also involve eradicating coexistent disease in the nose, sinuses or pharynx. Ideally the discharge is cleaned from the ear canal with suction under the operating microscope. Where these facilities are not available, gentle mopping may be performed. After cleaning, antibiotic–steroid drops are usually prescribed for a short period (see comments on p. 61). Cleaning may have to be done on a regular basis, and the importance of thorough cleaning must be emphasised, as drops will not be able to penetrate the middle ear if the canal is full of debris. Systemic antibiotic chemotherapy is not usually required. This treatment regimen should render the active mucosal disease inactive.

Surgical treatment should be considered in a number of specific situations:

- If the ear refuses to dry up, in spite of adequate local treatment, the possibility of continuing disease in the mastoid requiring surgical control should be borne in mind. In these patients a procedure to repair the eardrum (myringoplasty) may be combined with a cortical mastoidectomy to eradicate mucosal disease in the mastoid.
- If there is an aural polyp consisting of oedematous middle ear mucosa prolapsing through a perforation, this may need to be surgically removed if the ear is to settle.
- If the ear discharges intermittently the patient may be offered a myringoplasty procedure to repair the hole. This will allow the patient to get water in the ear with impunity and prevent the episodes of aural discharge with upper respiratory infections. Although hearing improvement is not the primary goal of such surgery, the hearing is frequently better afterwards. If it is not, this is likely to be because of damage to the ossicular chain by the chronic disease. It must be stressed that myringoplasty is usually elective and the underlying disease is not dangerous. Some patients therefore, especially if discharge is infrequent, prefer the alternative of using drops when the ear discharges, keeping water out of the ear and using a hearing aid to relieve any hearing difficulty. Operation is generally advisable for any ear which is troublesome, especially in healthy patients who are young, and would otherwise expect many years of nuisance and inconvenience, combined with potentially increasing damage to hearing.

Closure of the perforation can be accomplished in several different ways, depending upon size and position. A very small perforation may be treated in the outpatient department by 'freshening' the edges with a needle and covering the hole with a small patch of paper. Slightly larger perforations can be repaired using a plug of fat taken from the earlobe. Most patients, however, need a formal repair of the defect. The operation is a form of tympanoplasty – repair of the drum and ossicular chain. When the drum alone is repaired the procedure is a myringoplasty; when the ossicular chain alone is repaired this is an ossiculoplasty. The patient's own temporalis fascia is used to repair the drum, while ossicular chain defects may be repaired with the patient's own tissue (for example, one of the ossicles may be repositioned) or artificial materials such as hydroxyapatite. All these operations are microsurgical and require an advanced degree of surgical skill if consistently good results are to be obtained.

Inactive squamous epithelial chronic otitis media: retraction pocket Retraction pockets and atelectasis have been discussed above (p. 30). When they are 'inactive' there is no aural discharge and examination of the pocket under the microscope reveals a clean, dry pocket. Sometimes the limits of the pocket cannot be seen; an angled (30° or 70°) Hopkins rod telescope may be useful for looking round a corner towards the fundus of the pocket.

Active squamous epithelial chronic otitis media: cholesteatoma It is believed that acquired cholesteatoma often develops from such retraction pockets. Once adhesions form between the undersurface of a pocket and the middle ear contents, the pocket is unlikely to recover even if middle ear ventilation is re-established: they remain as collapsed areas in the attic or posterior segment of the pars tensa. The keratinising squamous epithelium of the drum normally throws off its dead layer of cells and no accumulation of debris occurs, but when a pocket forms and the normal self-cleaning process fails, keratin debris builds up within it and eventually becomes a true cholesteatoma (Fig. 4.6). Extrusion of the epithelium through the narrow neck of the sac becomes increasingly difficult and the lesion expands. The drum is not 'perforated' in the true sense of the word: the hole one sees is really the small, narrow opening of what can be a very large flask-like retraction pocket, the 'flask' itself being full of wax-like epithelial debris.

Other theories of cholesteatoma formation postulate that squamous metaplasia of the middle ear mucosa occurs in response to a chronic infection, or that there is ingrowth of squamous epithelium around the edges of a perforation, espe-

Otoscopic views in cases of cholesteatoma

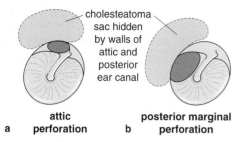

cholesteatoma sac hidden by walls of attic and posterior ear canal

a **attic perforation**   b **posterior marginal perforation**

Cross-section of right eardrum

cholesteatoma enveloping ossicles

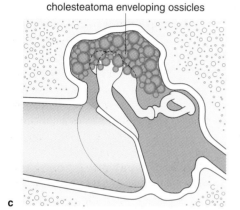

c

Fig. 4.6 Otoscopic view of tympanic membrane (a) and (b) and sagittal section (c) in cases of cholesteatoma. The full extent of the disease is outlined (dotted line) and is related to an attic (a) and marginal (b) perforation.

cially in cases of marginal perforation. It has also been suggested that ingrowth of basal cells, from the outer layer of the attic part of the drum into persisting submucous tissues within the attic spaces, may occur. It is possible that each of these mechanisms plays a part.

Bone destruction is a feature of acquired cholesteatoma, probably resulting from enzymatic activity in the subepithelial layers. Cholesterol granuloma has no relationship to cholesteatoma, although the names are confusing and the two conditions may coexist in the middle ear or mastoid. Cholesterol granuloma is caused by the presence of cholesterol crystals from a previous serosanguineous exudate. The crystals lead to a foreign body-type reaction, with the characteristic giant cells and granulomatous tissue.

Mention must be made of congenital cholesteatomas. These are primary inclusions of squamous epithelium within the temporal bone, usually at the apex, and are rare. By definition the drum must be intact for the diagnosis to be made. They produce extensive destruction and are usually only diagnosed when cranial nerves are affected. They are often closely related to the internal carotid artery and the jugular bulb. Computerised tomography (CT) and magnetic resonance imaging (MRI) can be useful in diagnosis, especially in distinguishing these lesions from others at the petrous apex. Their removal calls for advanced neuro-otological techniques.

The patient with aural discharge, hearing loss and 'atticoantral', 'unsafe' disease must be presumed to have a cholesteatoma until proven otherwise. As with mucosal chronic otitis media, the initial management consists of cleaning the ear under the operating microscope and treating it with antibiotic–steroid drops. Cholesteatomatous debris coming from a 'perforation' may then be evident. Clinical examination should include tests for potential complications, such as tuning fork and Barany box testing for conductive or sensorineural hearing loss and testing for the fistula sign. In some cases of cholesteatoma the disease causes erosion of the bone of the labyrinth. The most frequent site for such a fistula is the horizontal semicircular canal where it lies in the floor of the aditus. If such a fistula is present, any change of pressure in the middle ear will probably produce giddiness and nystagmus. The test is described on page 18. If a positive test is discovered it is an indication for urgent surgery because the labyrinth must still be functioning to some degree. Delay may allow labyrinthitis, and all that that entails, to ensue.

Hearing levels must be determined by audiometry, being especially careful to use appropriate masking in case the ear is 'dead'.

The role of radiology in the management of cholesteatoma has become somewhat controversial. Although the diagnosis is essentially a clinical one, CT of the ear provides the surgeon with valuable information about its anatomy and is particularly useful if complications are suspected or revision surgery is planned.

There are four principles of treatment:

- eradication of disease
- prevention of recurrence
- prevention of complications
- restoration of function.

Conservative treatment is of minimal value. Microsuction occasionally removes all diseased tissue and the ear may heal if the disease happens to be limited. There may be a role for such treatment in the very elderly and infirm or as a precursor to more definitive treatment.

Surgery aims to eliminate potentially dangerous disease. Preservation of hearing is important but not at the expense of compromised disease eradication and improvement in hearing (that is, restoration of hearing to normal or near normal levels). Surgery aims to give the patient a dry, stable, trouble-free ear; with modern surgical techniques this is possible in nearly all patients.

Eradication of disease is achieved with the primary surgical procedure. Any reconstructive surgery may be undertaken as a separate operation after an interval of several months, once the ear is safe and dry. Excision of the area of osteitis and cholesteatoma may require a relatively limited or an extensive surgical procedure: the extent is not usually known at the outset. Disease confined to the attic may be treated with an atticotomy. If it extends to the antrum an atticoantrostomy is created. When disease extends widely into the mastoid some form of mastoidectomy is required.

In a radical mastoidectomy the middle ear and mastoid cavities are thrown into one space by removal of the posterior wall of the external auditory canal as far down as the facial nerve will allow. Such a 'wall down' procedure exteriorises the mastoid segment and creates an open mastoid cavity. A classical radical mastoidectomy is in fact seldom carried out now; it involves removal of the malleus and incus as well as the drum remnant. Instead, if this sort of surgery is being carried out it is more usual to perform a modified radical mastoidectomy. The ossicles are preserved as far as possible and the drum remnant is retained (usually augmented by a graft) to close the middle ear and eustachian tube in order to prevent leakage of mucus into the cavity.

'Wall down' techniques of this type have stood the test of time and are known to provide a high degree of safety for the patient, but they also create their own problems. In particular, the presence of the cavity can itself be a considerable disability. Even the most stable mastoid cavity needs to be examined by an otologist once a year, and its owner often has to be careful about swimming and showering, etc. Other cavities become unstable from time to time and require treatment to dry them again. A significant proportion of cavities never epithelialise satisfactorily and are constantly moist.

The otologist who has found it necessary to carry out a 'wall down' procedure, in order to be as sure as possible of eradicating the disease, may therefore decide on some form of obliteration or of rebuilding procedure. A high degree of skill and judgement is required because even the most experienced surgeon may accidentally bury a microscopic area of residual disease which can later cause recurrence of cholesteatoma.

In recent years 'wall up' techniques, in which every attempt is made to eradicate disease completely while retaining intact the posterior bony canal wall and thereby avoiding the presence of an open mastoid cavity, have again become popular. In this combined approach technique the surgeon works partly permeatally and partly transmastoid, and in order to improve access creates a window from the mastoid to the posterior mesotympanum (a posterior tympanotomy). In the short term the outcome is very attractive, in that the patient has normal anatomy, no mastoid cavity and sometimes an excellent level of hearing. Unfortunately it is necessary to perform a second-look procedure 6–12 months after the initial surgery to check that no residual disease has inadvertently been left behind. The expectation is that by this time any residual disease will have grown sufficiently to be visible and removable. If no disease is present at this second procedure, any necessary ossicular reconstructive work can be undertaken. Alternatively, residual disease can be removed and the process of delay and re-exploration repeated, or a standard modified radical procedure can be performed. Although there is a place for combined approach 'canal wall up' procedures, it is limited by problems with a high incidence of recurrent disease. The technique should be applied to carefully selected patients.

Reconstruction of the hearing mechanism

Reconstruction of the hearing mechanism may be considered following treatment of both mucosal and cholesteatomatous types of chronic suppurative otitis media, or indeed in healed otitis media where parts of the ossicular chain are missing. Sometimes, however, the situation is such that any attempt at hearing reconstruction is contraindicated. For example, at one extreme no hearing improvement should be expected if there is severe degree of sensorineural loss combined with poor eustachian tube function, extensive destruction of the ossicles and perhaps only a small remnant of tympanic membrane remaining. The focus in such an ear should be on getting the ear dry, rather than on futile attempts to improve hearing. Conversely, in the case of a small perforation with a competent eustachian tube, normal middle ear mucosa and an intact ossicular chain, a good functional result is to be expected from closing the hole in the drum. If part of the ossicular chain were missing in such a case, once the drum had been repaired it would probably be reasonable to reconstruct the ossicular chain.

Surgical skill and experience are important factors in influencing the functional result of surgery, but the following are also important:

- Level of sensorineural reserve.
- Adequacy of eustachian tube function
- Quality of middle ear mucosa. Whereas the previous factors are outside the surgeon's control, the condition of the middle ear mucosa can be improved by treating sources of infection medically and surgically.
- Presence of an intact tympanic ring. This is an advantage in supporting the new drum.
- Feasibility of providing for adequate sound transmission. This implies the passage of vibration from the drum to the oval window across the closed, air-containing, mucosa-lined middle ear, and the provision of adequate

sound protection of the round window in order to produce a differential between the two windows.

Various materials and techniques have been employed for the purposes of reconstructing the drum and ossicles. Temporalis fascia, applied as an underlay graft to the medial surface of the tympanic membrane, is the usual grafting material for perforations. Perichondrium may also be used. The most common ossicular problem is that of a necrosed incus. Some form of strut can be placed between the malleus handle and stapes in these circumstances. The patient's own incus can be removed, remodelled with a drill and reinserted for this purpose. The problems of ossicular reconstruction become more complex with increasing degrees of destruction of the ossicular chain. In some patients only the malleus and footplate of the stapes may be present. In such cases a bony or artificial columella can be inserted between the remnants. The prostheses used for all these reconstructions are types of partial ossicular replacement prosthesis ('PORP'). Even more complex is the situation in which the malleus is absent. In this case a total ossicular replacement prosthesis (TORP) – drum to footplate – may be needed.

TUBERCULOSIS OF THE EAR

This disease occurs mainly in children and is insidious in onset; widespread bone disease may be present but with little outward evidence. Infection is secondary to disease elsewhere and usually reaches the ear via the eustachian tube by infiltration of its mucosa. In adults infectious material may pass up the lumen. Haematogenous spread also occurs.

In countries where tuberculosis remains common, or in a patient with known tuberculosis, a chronic ear infection with many beefy granulations may arouse suspicion; sometimes a complication such as facial palsy will raise the possibility. Biopsy will give the diagnosis. In such patients surgical treatment should be as conservative as possible. Treatment is primarily medical; the ear heals as the patient's systemic disease is brought under control.

NON-SUPPURATIVE DISEASES OF THE MIDDLE EAR

Healed otitis media (adhesive hearing loss)

This type of hearing loss is caused by fibrosis and necrosis of the mucosa, ossicles and ligaments of the middle ear. Sometimes the disorder may take the form of a fibrocystic obliteration of the middle ear cleft. It is essentially the end result of healed infection, which may have been either overt or such as to have passed almost unnoticed at the time. Antibiotics may have helped to mask the continuing damage. In some patients there is no history of previous ear trouble and the condition must therefore be regarded as a result of chronic infection in the nasopharynx which has produced recurring tubotympanitis.

Clinically the slowly progressive conductive hearing loss is often bilateral; the drum is thickened and opaque and generally reduced in mobility, corresponding to the changes within the middle ear cleft. Tympanosclerosis is the name given to a somewhat similar disorder in which chalk-like deposits occur in the drum and middle ear mucosa, with fixation of the ossicular chain.

Tympanotomy can be considered if the sensorineural reserve is adequate; limited adhesions can sometimes be divided or bypassed using techniques similar to those in tympanoplasty. The result of the operation usually depends on the extent of the damage and is often disappointing. If the hearing loss is severe enough, a hearing aid can be considered and generally the result will be better than with operation.

Otitic barotrauma

This can result from any circumstance associated with increasing external pressure, such as tunnelling and diving, but is seen most frequently after flying. To maintain an equal pressure on both sides of the intact eardrum, a normally functioning eustachian tube is essential. The movements of swallowing allow the tube to open momentarily, but if patency is disturbed by nasopharyngeal disease (most commonly a cold), the mechanism may fail.

Ascent, i.e. decompression, is generally without discomfort, as air can escape readily down the eustachian tube. On descent, however, especially if it is rapid, frequent and determined efforts at swallowing or performing the Valsalva manoeuvre may fail to clear the tube. This results in the persistence of the low pressure in the middle ear, often with collapse of the drum and accumulation of fluid. There may be bleeding into the ear. Severe pain and conductive hearing loss can occur.

The established condition may be readily relieved by aerating the middle ear cleft. This can be done most effectively and most speedily by a quick paracentesis. The patient then attempts the Valsalva manoeuvre, or alternatively the fluid can be cleared with a pneumatic speculum. A formal myringotomy is not indicated. Eustachian tube catheterisation is a less effective alternative. The strictest sterile precautions should be observed and antibiotic cover should be provided in view of the likelihood of nasopharyngeal infection.

Although the term 'otitic barotrauma' generally refers to the condition described above, it must also be noted that pressure change can sometimes produce labyrinthine rupture, with perhaps the creation of a perilymph fistula at the oval or round window. This produces a sensorineural type of hearing loss, which is generally severe and demands immediate recognition if a permanent and severe sensorineural hearing loss is to be avoided. Unfortunately, such patients are often seen too late because they have been misdiagnosed as having a conductive hearing loss caused by middle ear effusion. The negative Rinne is in fact a false-negative. Perilymph fistula is further discussed on page 60.

Exposure to noise incidental to flying can cause hearing changes of cochlear type due to temporary threshold shift (p. 61).

Otosclerosis

This is a progressive disease that, as a rule, causes symptoms early in adult life. Occasionally it is found in quite young patients and tends to present more frequently in the female – there is a familial tendency. The hearing loss may progress almost to total deafness, but in the more severe cases a sensorineural hearing loss will be found to have supervened. The condition is commonly bilateral.

Hearing loss is the chief symptom. There may be some tinnitus; occasionally this can be severe. Giddiness may also occur but is rarely a disability. Characteristically the patient speaks in a quiet voice in sharp contradistinction to the harsh unmodulated tones of those with sensorineural hearing loss. Not infrequently patients are conscious that they hear better in a noisy environment: this is known as *paracusis Willisi,* and it is marked in early cases. It is a result of the fact that in otosclerosis the patient hears ambient noise less well, whereas people with normal hearing automatically raise their voice to overcome background noise, and the otosclerotic patient thus enjoys a comparative advantage. Paracusis may be found in other kinds of conductive hearing loss but is characteristic of otosclerosis.

Inspection of the ears usually shows the drums to be normal. Rinne's test is negative and Weber is usually lateralised to the more affected ear. In advanced cases there may be sensorineural hearing loss, which can be severe and which is associated with masses of otosclerotic bone occurring around the cochlea. Such hearing loss can be assessed accurately only by audiometric testing. None of the various explanatory theories is satisfactory.

The disease is caused by the laying down of spongy bone of a vascular type around the oval window (Fig. 4.7). New bone may also be formed on the cochlear side of the oval window. The immediate effect is fixation of the stapes (Fig. 4.8). Otosclerotic foci usually occur at multiple sites in the labyrinthine capsule. The aetiology remains obscure. Most authorities agree that there is a genetic factor; hormonal influences play a part, and the disease often begins during pregnancy.

The choice of treatment lies between the use of a hearing aid and operation. Modern hearing aids are extremely satisfactory for patients with a conductive type of hearing loss, and especially for patients with otosclerosis. Their use is comparatively free from complications, apart from occasional breakdowns and exhausted batteries, so some patients opt for a hearing aid.

The alternative is surgical treatment. This will be preferred by many patients, especially younger ones,

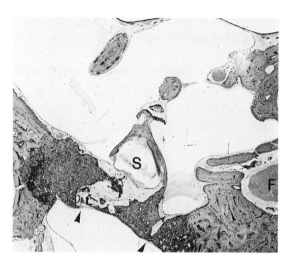

Fig. 4.7 Otosclerosis. Transverse section of the middle ear at the level of the oval window. The edges of the oval window are arrowed. New bone has grown over this area and has entirely immobilised the stapes (S). F, facial nerve. Photograph courtesy of Prof. H. Schuknecht.

a Immobilised footplate caused by otosclerosis

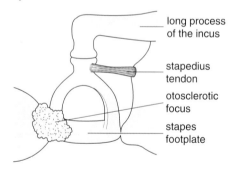

long process of the incus

stapedius tendon

otosclerotic focus

stapes footplate

b Stapedectomy

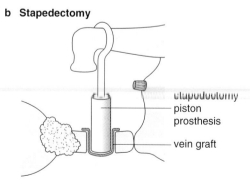

stapedotomy piston prosthesis

vein graft

Fig. 4.8 Stapedectomy.

who do not wish to be seen with a hearing aid.

The first successful operation was fenestration of the lateral semicircular canal, but it had a number of disadvantages. Stapedectomy is the modern treatment. Although this operation requires a great deal of skill and experience in microsurgical techniques, it is not a serious procedure as far as the patient is concerned, and can be done under either local or general anaesthesia. The drum is elevated and folded forwards, and the diagnosis of stapes fixation is confirmed by the use of a suitable probe to palpate the ossicle. There are several forms of this operation. The head, neck and crura of the stapes are removed, and a small opening is then made in the middle of the central part of the footplate. A piston-like prosthesis is inserted to restore ossicular mobility. Its tip just protrudes through the opening in the footplate; its hook is clamped on to the incus (Fig. 4.8). Stapedectomy requires a high degree of microsurgical skill if good results are to be obtained consistently and disasters avoided.

After stapedectomy the disturbance to the patient is generally minimal. Giddiness is slight and usually settles in a few days. Improvement in hearing is fairly rapid, and in about 90% of patients a competent surgeon will expect to bring the hearing up to the level of the patient's cochlear reserve; in another 8% the hearing will be lifted part of the way up to this level; in about 1 or 2% deterioration of hearing occurs. In these 1 or 2% a sensorineural hearing loss develops, the cause of which is not always clear. This risk is a small one but must always be mentioned to patients because it usually makes the wearing of a hearing aid impossible in the operated ear. It is a complication that can occasionally occur even in the most experienced hands but is undoubtedly related to an individual surgeon's skill. For this reason each surgeon must audit his or her results and be able to tell the patient the likelihood of this complication occurring.

Perilymph fistula is a complication of stapedectomy which must be mentioned. It occasionally arises as a late complication and is characterised by a sudden fall in hearing; the hearing loss is of sensorineural type. Some temporary recovery may occur spontaneously, but further episodes of sudden impairment usually occur until eventually a total sensorineural deafness results. If this complication is recognised early, an urgent revision operation is called for in an attempt to salvage whatever hearing remains. Regrettably, the complication is too frequently misdiagnosed as 'catarrhal' hearing loss, and by the time the patient is seen by a specialist the sensorineural loss is irreversible.

MIDDLE EAR INJURIES
Penetrating injuries

Penetrating injuries of the ear may occur if a twig or a hairgrip is accidentally pushed into the ear. The tympanic membrane may be perforated and the ossicular chain disrupted (p. 29).

Fractures of the temporal bone

In *longitudinal fractures* the line runs in the axis of the external meatus. The tympanic ring is broken and the drum and roof of the meatus are torn. There is bleeding from the ear, and hearing loss of conductive type. The laceration is frequently obscured by blood clot and swelling. Longitudinal fractures account for about 80% of temporal bone fractures; fortunately the inner ear is not involved and facial paralysis is unusual. If paralysis occurs, it is generally late, as a result of swelling, and carries a good prognosis.

In *transverse fractures* the line is anteroposterior. The tympanic ring is spared. The inner ear is often in the line of fracture, so complete loss of function is the rule. Examination of the tympanic membrane shows a bluish, bulging appearance caused by the presence of blood in the middle ear. When the patient regains consciousness, it will be found that there is total sensorineural hearing loss, as well as nystagmus and giddiness caused by the destruction of the vestibular labyrinth, which will gradually compensate with the passage of time. Approximately 50% of patients have a facial paralysis. The lesion is generally severe and may be at any level, including the labyrinthine segment or even internal meatus. In mixed types of fracture dural laceration and cerebrospinal fluid (CSF) otorrhoea may occur.

Treatment is generally conservative. The ear should be protected with a sterile dressing and systemic antibiotics given: on no account should it be syringed. If infection occurs, it is treated on the usual lines but a special watch should be maintained for intracranial spread, and if a chronic infection is already present it may be eliminated by the appropriate mastoid operation as soon as the patient is sufficiently recovered.

Facial palsy may require surgical treatment, especially if early and severe, because in such patients the lesion is inevitably a serious one. The timing of exploration depends on the patient's head injuries and general injuries. Facial palsy occurring late only rarely requires exploration of the nerve. Hearing loss caused by involvement of the cochlea in the fracture line is not amenable to treatment. Conductive hearing loss generally recovers spontaneously, but, if it persists, investigation of the middle ear is indicated, via a tympanotomy a few months later. Dislocation of the incus may be present, and can be corrected surgically. Cerebrospinal fluid leakage must be treated by appropriate chemotherapy in the first instance; it will nearly always cease spontaneously after a few days. Healing of the fracture line, however, is only by fibrous union, and such a patient may be at risk of future meningitis at any time from otitis media. Accordingly, it is preferable to arrange for a more secure repair, using a neurosurgical middle fossa extradural approach for the insertion of a graft of fascia lata to reinforce the injured area.

MIDDLE EAR TUMOURS

Paragangliomas (glomus tumours) arise from the glomus bodies which occur normally at various body sites, including the promontory and the jugular bulb. Early paragangliomas produce a pulsatile tinnitus as a result of their vascularity and can be seen pulsating behind the intact eardrum. Larger ones protrude as polyps in the ear canal. Although histologically they may be classed as benign tumours, they present serious problems in treatment, particularly if they are large, on account of their vascularity and anatomical relationships. This is true especially of those of jugular origin, which tend to be invasive, arise actually within the wall of the jugular bulb, and not infrequently involve its lumen and adjacent skull base (Fig. 4.9).

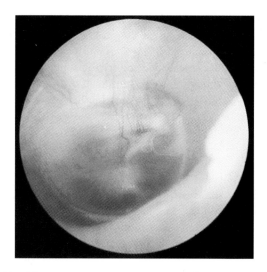

Fig. 4.9 A glomus tumour is visible behind the posteroinferior quadrant of the tympanic membrane.

Carcinoma also may occur in the ear. It is usually a complication of many years of uncontrolled suppuration, either in the ear or following persistent discharge from a mastoid cavity. The onset of pain is the symptom which usually causes the patient to seek advice. Combined irradiation and surgery is the usual treatment, but is often disappointing, although in certain cases radical excision of the petrous bone can be curative even when previous radiotherapy and surgery have failed to control the disease.

> ### ► Key points
>
> - ► The ear should be kept dry in cases of tympanic membrane perforation.
> - ► Retraction pockets result from negative middle ear pressure and may develop into cholesteatoma.
> - ► 'Safe' perforations should be distinguished from potentially 'unsafe' perforations.
> - ► Recurrent aural discharge requires investigation.
> - ► Otitis media with effusion ('glue ear') is extremely common in childhood.
> - ► Patients with suspected cholesteatoma require specialist management.
> - ► Otosclerosis is a common cause of conductive hearing loss with a normal eardrum.

Complications of otitis media

5

INTRODUCTION

The complications of otitis media (Fig. 5.1) are seen less frequently now than in the past, probably because of the increased use of antibiotic chemotherapy. They are still however extremely important and may be life threatening. The following classical clinical descriptions are reproduced to remind clinicians who may only rarely see these conditions. Prompt treatment is essential and can only occur once the condition has been correctly diagnosed.

Acute mastoiditis

Acute mastoiditis is a complication of acute otitis media, and in its classical form is now a rare disease in most Western countries: it is nevertheless not uncommon in those countries where access to medical facilities is more limited. More frequent in children than in adults, it is due to extension of an acute otitis media into what was previously a normal, pneumatised, cellular mastoid. It cannot occur in an acellular, sclerotic type of mastoid. Acute infection *can* be superimposed on a chronic attico-antral type of infection in which the cholesteatoma has invaded the mastoid segment, but the term 'acute mastoiditis' is not normally applied in this situation.

    Some degree of inflammatory reaction within the mastoid frequently accompanies acute otitis media. Its extent is determined by several factors,

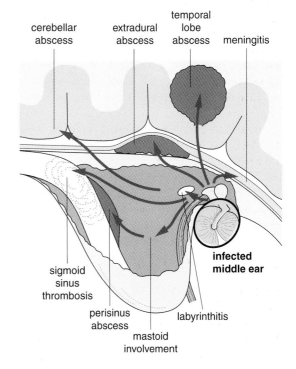

Fig. 5.1 Complications of middle ear infection showing directions of spread.

including the cellularity of the mastoid, the anatomy of the aditus and the virulence of the infection. Swelling of the lining of the aditus may prevent proper drainage of infection in the mastoid area and accelerate destruction of bone cells. Continuous hyperaemia in the presence of infection causes decalcification of bone trabeculae, so that in advanced cases the whole area becomes one large cavity filled with pus and granulations. If the disease continues uncontrolled, the infection may break through towards the middle cranial fossa, the posterior fossa or the sigmoid sinus. In more fortunate cases the pus may break through the superficial cortex and form an abscess under the periosteum.

Although acute otitis media invariably precedes mastoiditis, this may not have been noticed. Evidence of it can, however, always be found. One of the outstanding signs of the onset of mastoiditis is pain. While pain is a feature of acute otitis media, after myringotomy or spontaneous perforation of the drum it tends to disappear in a few hours, or at the most after 3 or 4 days. If pain recurs or, not having completely disappeared, increases in severity, this is an indication of progressing mastoid infection. In these circumstances the pain may be in the ear, but it is more often located behind it in the mastoid bone. It may remain localised to one spot or radiate all over the side of the head in severe spasms.

With the onset of mastoiditis, aural discharge usually ceases or becomes more profuse. Cessation means that the membrane lining the aditus has become so swollen that the discharge is being dammed up in the mastoid cells. Relief by mastoid operation will almost certainly be required. Increased discharge suggests the further involvement of mastoid cells by infection.

A rise of temperature usually accompanies the spread of infection, but in uncomplicated mastoiditis the temperature rarely rises above 38.5°C. Sharp rises above this suggest further complications, in particular blood infection. Generally speaking, temperature is an unreliable guide to the condition within the mastoid cells, as many a case of advanced suppuration is afebrile. A more reliable indication of the course of an infection can be obtained by the careful observation of the pulse rate. This is especially true in the case of children. A slowly rising pulse rate is always a danger sign, and may of itself constitute sufficient reason for operation. Conversely, sudden and unexplained fall without corresponding fall of temperature must always arouse suspicion of intracranial complication. Where mastoid involvement is suspected, a patient must never be considered out of danger until the pulse rate has fallen to normal.

In the majority of cases the onset of mastoiditis is accompanied by increased hearing loss. The general appearance of the patient must always be taken into account – with the rise of temperature the patient appears flushed and has an anxious look; the tongue, in most cases, is heavily coated. There is increasing tenderness over the mastoid area. This is most marked in front of and behind the mastoid tip, but may spread all over the bone. In infants the tenderness is frequently found over the mastoid antrum, as the mastoid process itself may not yet be developed. If careful search is made over the mastoid area, thickening of the periosteum will be detected. This is most easily found by standing behind the patient with one hand on each mastoid, carefully comparing the sensation when palpating the bone. On the sound side the bony outline is clear and the root of the zygoma and meatal spine are distinct. On the affected side there is a feeling that a thin sheet of rubber overlies the bone. As the condition worsens, these signs are more noticeable. There is increasing oedema of the overlying skin and tissues, which is initially found over the mastoid antrum and the posterior wall of the external meatus. When fully developed the swelling has a characteristic appearance: the auricle is pushed outwards and downwards by the oedema and the subperiosteal accumulation of pus, while the skinfold behind the auricle is preserved. There is still tenderness over the bone on deep pressure. If the external meatus is examined, the condition will be seen to differ from normal in that there appears to be a narrowing of the meatus. If this is examined closely, the narrowing will be found to be caused by depression of the roof of the meatus. The sagging appears to commence at the drum membrane, giving the passage a funnel shape.

In the majority of cases a perforation is seen in the drum membrane, through which pus is flowing or pulsating. It must be borne in mind, however, that mastoiditis may occur where the drum membrane appears to be intact. In some cases the pus may burrow along the posterior meatal wall under the periosteum and finally perforate the posterior wall of the auditory canal. At first the symptoms closely resemble furunculosis. A swelling is seen on the posterior wall, from which pus is oozing, but owing to the oedema no view can be obtained of the drum. Before a diagnosis can be made, other points such as the position of pain and tenderness, and pain on movement of the auricle, must be considered. The state of the hearing, the tuning fork tests and radiographs are also important.

The differential diagnosis between mastoiditis and those conditions closely simulating it should be considered. Confusion may arise with a number of conditions, but of these the chief are furunculosis, otitis externa and erysipelas. The points of similarity are pain and discharge from the ear and oedema of the tissues surrounding the auricle. In some cases there is hearing loss. The difference between mastoiditis and one of the other conditions may be so slight as to give even an experienced clinician great difficulty in diagnosis. It must constantly be remembered that an otitis externa or furunculosis may coexist with an acute or subacute otitis media. The presence of discharge in the external meatus may have set up the external irritation which was responsible for the otitis externa, and it is in these cases that the greatest difficulties arise. The most certain method of making the diagnosis is by examining the drum membrane. If this is normal there can be no otitis media or mastoiditis. Sometimes, however, it is impossible to see the drum, and experience shows that it is in such cases that mistakes are most common.

CT of the mastoid may demonstrate soft tissue density in the middle ear and/or mastoid. This may be pus but could equally be swollen soft tissues. Conversely, air may be present and this effectively excludes the diagnosis. Complications of mastoiditis, especially abscess formation in adjacent areas, may be seen. Plain radiographs of the mastoid may be useful, especially if CT is not available. Comparison of the two sides may demonstrate abscess formation.

Masked mastoiditis

Masked or 'silent' mastoiditis has replaced traditional acute mastoiditis in many parts of the world. The disease is 'masked' because of the antibiotics that have been used to treat the infection, often suboptimally. It should be suspected in those children who are subject to repeated episodes of acute otitis media going on to otorrhoea, and in whom the ear does not easily become dry and normal with conventional and apparently adequate treatment. During an attack, aching pain is felt in or behind the ear; there may be a temporary increase in hearing loss and there may be transient discharge. The picture differs in small degree from that of otitis media, although there may be more mastoid tenderness. The main difference is that the ear and hearing do not return to normal and mild exacerbations continue to occur.

Between attacks a degree of conductive hearing loss persists, the drum remains dull, immobile and featureless. Tenderness and periosteal oedema over the mastoid are usually absent.

The condition is diagnosed partly by the ability to recognise these unusual signs and partly radiologically. Soft tissue density is seen within the mastoid on CT; on plain radiographs clouding of the mastoid cells is seen. Treatment is by a cortical (Schwartze) mastoidectomy. The bone is abnormally soft and the mastoid cells filled with thickened mucosa and exudate.

Zygomatic mastoiditis

The zygoma may be so extensively pneumatised that the infection may extend forwards and thus appear to cause swelling and tenderness in front of, and above, the auditory meatus.

Bezold's mastoiditis

Another form of extension, known as Bezold's mastoiditis, is the condition in which a large tip cell gives way and the pus extends downwards into the sheath of the sternomastoid muscle.

Treatment of mastoiditis

Intensive treatment with appropriate antibiotics can reverse the early stages of acute mastoiditis. Care must be taken not to produce a masked mastoiditis instead, however, and resolution must be complete. In case of doubt, it is wiser to operate rather than delay and risk loss of hearing, incomplete resolution and potential complications.

The operation to treat acute mastoiditis is the cortical (Schwartze) mastoidectomy (p. 57). The aims of the operation are to provide drainage of sepsis, prevent its extension and preserve hearing. Since the patient's safety is paramount, timely intervention and adequate surgical drainage is essential. Once hearing is lost over a period, some loss will remain. The longer an infected area is allowed to drain through the middle ear, the less likely an eventual return to full function. The results of surgery are excellent and full recovery of hearing may normally be expected.

Labyrinthitis

Labyrinthitis continues to be an unusual although not particularly rare complication of acute or chronic otitis media, but it is significant because it may be a precursor of meningitis. Early recognition and urgent treatment help preserve function and prevent further spread of infection. Infection can develop after erosion of the bony capsule of the labyrinth; it may occur through vascular channels or by surgical injury to the lateral semicircular canal or the footplate of the stapes in the course of operation. Rarely, it can occur as an infection from primary meningitis.

Erosion of the bone of the labyrinth may expose the membranous labyrinth to infection from the middle ear. This is caused most frequently by cholesteatoma, usually in the horizontal semicircular canal, and may result in repeated attacks of a localised serous inflammation known as 'circumscribed' labyrinthitis. Infection by this route, as by any other, may eventually become widespread. Such diffuse labyrinthitis may initially be of a serous nature, but can later become purulent.

When the infection settles down, one of two things happens: either the pus becomes organised and the labyrinth fills with bone, or pus becomes locked up within the labyrinth. This stage is called 'latent' labyrinthitis.

In addition to symptoms already present as a result of middle ear disease, symptoms and signs caused by labyrinthine irritation and failure become evident. These consist of giddiness, loss of balance, vomiting and nystagmus, as well as increased hearing loss. This further hearing impairment is of the sensorineural type.

When giddiness is intense, the patient often adopts a characteristic attitude in bed, lying on the sound side and looking towards the affected ear, because in that position the giddiness and nystagmus are greatly lessened.

Level of hearing depends on the stage of infection. The primary infection in the ear may have already produced considerable hearing loss of conductive type – any hearing loss caused by the labyrinthitis will be of sensorineural type. The fistula sign should be sought; if it is present it means that the labyrinth is exposed but also that it is still functioning. In a diagnosis of acute labyrinthitis, caloric tests should not be carried out as they may initiate spread of infection to the meninges. As the disease advances, all signs of function will be lost. The negative Rinne now becomes a false-negative; tuning fork and noise box testing indicate a dead ear. In latent labyrinthitis full compensation will have been completed by the time the patient is first seen, but the proper use of the noise box with the tuning fork tests will enable the presence of a dead ear to be identified.

Antibiotics should be given in full dosage when labyrinthitis is suspected, as it may be arrested at any stage with energetic and appropriate treatment of the middle ear infection. Return of function depends on the speed and efficiency of treatment, provided that inflammation has not already caused severe damage within the labyrinth.

In the early stages of serous labyrinthitis, if the patient is kept in bed with the head immobilised between pillows the nystagmus may be expected to subside within a few days, and when it has settled the appropriate mastoid operation should be carried out urgently. Fairly urgent operation should also be performed on those patients with symptoms of labyrinthine irritation who are found to have a positive fistula sign. The most likely site of a fistula is on the horizontal semicircular canal, as previously mentioned.

When a fistula has been identified, the surgeon must decide how to deal with it. There is no unanimity on this point if hearing is still present, and with any method of management there is risk of a dead ear occurring even though the utmost gentleness has been employed. One method is to leave undisturbed a thin layer of cholesteatomatous membrane over the fistula. In this case the fistula must be exteriorised by making an open type of mastoid cavity. Alternatively, the cholesteatoma can be carefully lifted off and the exposed fistula covered with a graft of temporalis fascia. Either way the utmost care is necessary.

Another management problem occurs in patients in whom the disease has already produced a dead ear, that is, when the latent stage has been reached. In the course of the operation to eradicate the chronic otitis media, the surgeon must decide whether to leave alone a labyrinth that may still contain pus or whether to explore it. In latent labyrinthitis the labyrinth spaces may have become obliterated with fibrous tissue or bone, or may be filled with pus, either infected or sterile. To leave a potentially infective condition in the ear is dangerous, and it is recommended that the labyrinth should be explored.

The outstanding danger in all patients with labyrinthitis is the complication of meningitis. A constant watch must be kept for this complication and a lumbar puncture carried out if it is suspected. The presence of pus in the CSF is an indication for surgical drainage of the labyrinth.

Loss of one labyrinth may cause difficulties in balance, especially in older people, and rehabilitation exercises under a competent physiotherapist will do much to hasten recovery.

Otitic septicaemia

Otitic septicaemia is typically associated with sinus thrombosis, and occasionally with an acute otitis or fulminating mastoiditis. In young children this may occur during epidemics of gastroenteritis. The patient is extremely ill and the temperature fluctuates wildly. Blood culture may or may not be positive. Owing to debilitation and malnutrition this disease is extremely dangerous and, while antibiotics must be used, intensive supportive measures are also required.

INTRACRANIAL COMPLICATIONS

Intracranial complications continue to occur and to be serious; some have significant morbidity and

mortality. In more fortunate patients the pus resulting from mastoiditis erodes laterally through the cortex to present as a fluctuant area overlying the mastoid. Sometimes the cortex is dense and pus will take the line of least resistance, travelling medially to produce intracranial complications (Fig. 5.1).

These complications are found more frequently in adults than in children, owing to the relative thickness of the cortex in adults and the firm union of the sutures. Infections caused by *Pneumococcus* spp. are particularly liable to complications. The complications are listed in Box 5.1.

> ■ Box 5.1
>
> **Intracranial complications of otitis media**
> - Perisinus abscess
> - Sigmoid (lateral) sinus thrombosis
> - Cavernous sinus thrombosis
> - Extradural abscess
> - Otogenic brain abscess
> - Meningitis

Perisinus abscess

The plate of bone covering the sigmoid (lateral) sinus may be eroded by prolonged suppuration. Any portion of the sinus in contact with the mastoid may be involved and the abscess may not be limited to the wall of the sigmoid sinus but can extend as part of an extradural abscess into the middle or posterior fossa. It may be wise, in the course of mastoidectomy for acute mastoiditis, to expose a small area of sigmoid sinus to ensure there is no perisinus pus, or indeed a sinus thrombosis. Perisinus abscess causes no characteristic symptoms but is important because it is a precursor of sigmoid sinus thrombosis. Treatment consists of the free drainage of the affected area by appropriate mastoid surgery. Bone should be removed until healthy dura is exposed around any areas of granulation.

Sigmoid (lateral) sinus thrombosis

Sigmoid sinus thrombosis is rare in Western countries. The granulation tissue that forms on the wall of the sigmoid sinus with a perisinus abscess offers considerable resistance to entry of infection into the lumen. Such spread enters by direct extension or retrograde thrombosis of veins passing into the sinus. Initially a mural clot may form but gradually this can build up to produce total occlusion and established sigmoid (lateral) sinus thrombosis. The extent and position of the thrombosis varies: it may extend upwards to the torcula or invade the superior sagittal or other sinuses. Downwards it may extend into the jugular bulb and, rarely, the internal jugular vein. The jugular bulb may be affected by direct extension through the floor of the middle ear. Formation of a healthy thrombus is a defence mechanism, but the thrombus may become infected, soften and break up, resulting in pyaemia and septicaemia.

The classical symptom in unmasked sigmoid sinus thrombosis is repeated rigors associated with sharp fluctuations in temperature. The rigor may last a few minutes, half an hour or longer; the temperature then rises rapidly to 39°C. These attacks usually come on in the evening, and by the next morning the temperature has fallen to normal or subnormal. The pulse rate remains rapid. During the rigor the patient looks anxious, grey and ill, but between attacks is well and feels fit. This is a deceptive stage and may delude the inexperienced into fatal delay.

The clinical picture may be confused because the patient has been given antibiotics. Rigors are frequently absent and the temperature only moderately elevated. The ear condition may appear to respond to treatment but the patient fails to show general improvement. The Tobey–Ayer test (below) may be helpful but a definitive diagnosis may only be possible by exploring the mastoid and aspirating the exposed sinus. Late signs of the disease include pyaemic abscesses, high white count and positive blood cultures, signs of raised intracranial pressure and thickening and tenderness over the line of the internal jugular vein.

The CSF (Tobey–Ayer) test may be useful. The CSF pressure is measured via a lumbar puncture. The jugular veins on each side are compressed in turn. Compression on the thrombosed side may produce little or no increase in pressure; on the unaffected side a much greater rise is seen.

The treatment of sinus thrombosis consists of opening the sinus and removing the infected clot. Superiorly, bone is removed until healthy-looking sinus has been exposed for about a centimetre. The sinus is then opened longitudinally and the septic clot removed until free bleeding occurs. Bleeding is readily controlled by inserting a pack of medicated ribbon gauze between the bone and sinus wall, compressing the lumen. Packing should preferably not be placed in the lumen, otherwise bleeding can restart when it is removed. The lower end of the sinus is dealt with in a similar manner as far as practicable. Anticoagulants are not normally given, but antibiotics are continued in full dosage according to bacteriological results.

Masked sinus thrombosis

The preceding account is based on the natural course of disease uncomplicated by antibiotic therapy. Antibiotics have caused the virtual disappearance of this clinical picture and diagnosis must be made on the basis of a knowledge of the fundamental character of the disease and the probable effects of antibiotic therapy. In the child, it is likely to follow acute mastoiditis; in the adult, to be the result of cholesteatoma infection. The features that are suppressed are the fever, rigors and infection of the bloodstream. Diagnosis usually depends on exploration of the mastoid and examination of the sinus.

Otitic intracranial hypertension

The old term 'otitic hydrocephalus' is misleading – most cases are idiopathic. There is no hydrocephalus, in the sense that there is no enlargement of the ventricles. Obstruction of venous outflow by an otogenic sinus thrombosis is not necessarily present. The cause of the high CSF pressure is not fully understood.

Headache, papilloedema and sometimes VIth nerve paralysis provide the clues to diagnosis. Papilloedema demands immediate relief by reduction in CSF pressure to prevent optic atrophy and blindness. This can usually be achieved by medical therapy using diuretics and steroids. Surgical decompression using a ventriculoperitoneal shunt may be necessary.

Extradural abscess

Disease may reach the middle or the posterior fossa by direct extension of infection, and an abscess may be formed, which may be extradural. This can be part of the mastoid abscess. The spread of inflammation and the absorption of bone in the mastoid areas can lead to infection and necrosis of the dural plate. The dural plate having given way, the dura mater is exposed to the infection, and a reaction takes place. There is a thickening of the membrane, granulations are formed upon the surface and the condition is then known as an extradural abscess. This type of abscess is frequently found in the middle fossa and may track back until it comes into contact with the sigmoid sinus. The posterior fossa may also be the site of an abscess. Such cases are usually an extension of a perisinus infection which burrows forward into Trautman's triangle posterior to the labyrinth.

This type of abscess may be suspected in patients suffering from headache with signs of early meningeal irritation, but is rarely diagnosed before surgery unless a scan has been done. An extradural abscess gives no specific symptoms or signs.

Brain abscesses

Otogenic brain abscess usually arises by direct extension through thrombophlebitis or via perivascular sheaths and is therefore adjacent to the temporal bone, into which a track often exists. Diagnosis may be obscured by coexistent complication, for example meningitis, caused by the traverse of the infection across several tissue planes on its way into the brain.

Most abscesses arise from chronic otitis on which an acute infection has been superimposed, and particularly from the type with cholesteatoma. Initially the lesion is a poorly defined encephalitis which gradually localises and encapsulates; treatment is accordingly planned to encourage encapsulation.

Metastatic abscesses from embolism are rare, often multiple and at a distance from the primary focus. Traumatic abscess can complicate a penetrating wound or a skull fracture in the presence of a chronic ear infection. The abscess enlarges mainly at the expense of the white matter; spread is thus towards the ventricle, into which fatal rupture can occur.

Brain abscess passes through the following stages: (1) initial invasion; (2) encephalitis; (3) a latent period; (4) a stage of increasing intracranial pressure; and (5) a terminal stage.

A long-standing otorrhoea may have diminished or ceased prior to the onset of symptoms, which can be considered under the following headings.

Systemic and cerebral infection

Chills or rigor may occur, with an initial rise in pulse rate and temperature and sometimes with vomiting and headaches. When the suppuration is established it may pass into the latent stage, in which it can remain for several weeks. During this period the patient may go on working and appear normal. It is common, however, for there to be some feeling of malaise, the occasional headache and vomiting. The temperature usually becomes subnormal and the pulse rate shows periodic slowing to perhaps 40–50 beats per minute. Epileptic fits are not unusual during this stage but are not of localising value unless of focal type.

Intracranial pressure

As the abscess absorbs more brain tissue, the surrounding oedema causes signs of cerebral compression: headache of great severity, occasional vomiting, periodic drop in pulse rate, and indefinite signs of meningeal irritation. Ocular changes – papilloedema and indefinite nystagmus – may be found but are not constant. Paresis of ocular muscles occurs but normally only in the terminal stages.

Focal symptoms

These are of theoretical interest only: to await their appearance is to invite disaster. Nominal aphasia is pathognomonic of an abscess in the left temporal lobe, provided the patient is right-handed. Contralateral paralysis is a comparatively uncommon symptom and is the result of pressure on the internal capsule or on the cortical motor area. Changes in visual field occur when the abscess is large, and may cause a homonymous hemianopia.

CT provides the most accurate and rapid method of diagnosing or excluding an abscess. It is rapid, non-invasive and can easily be repeated to follow the progress of an abscess. Lumbar puncture can be dangerous and misleading: CSF is under pressure and fatal coning may occur.

Cerebellar abscess is much less frequent than temporal lobe abscess. It is caused chiefly by the spread of infection from labyrinthitis, perisinus abscess or sinus thrombosis. Headache, vomiting, drowsiness and papilloedema may occur: general symptoms are as previously described. It should be noted, as in all subtentorial 'tumour' formation, that papilloedema in posterior fossa abscess occurs early.

Localising symptoms are those of the cerebellar syndrome and are homolateral. Ataxia, rombergism, dysdiadochokinesia, indistinct speech, atony of muscles, incoordination, skewed position of the head, increased reflexes on the affected side and clonus may be found. As with temporal lobe abscess, CT provides the most rapid and accurate method of diagnosis.

Treatment of brain abscesses

The treatment of brain abscesses is a specialised area and whenever possible neurosurgical advice and assistance should be obtained. Among the important issues to discuss are the type and duration of antibiotic chemotherapy, the timing and approach of the surgery to drain the abscess and the timing of the mastoid surgery to eradicate the underlying middle ear and mastoid disease.

Meningitis

Meningitis is inflammation of the covering membranes of the brain. We are mainly concerned here with inflammation of the pia-arachnoid (i.e. of the subarachnoid CSF-containing space). Infection may be: (1) through the labyrinth; (2) from sigmoid sinus thrombosis; (3) from blood vessels crossing the subarachnoid space; (4) occasionally by rupture of a brain abscess into either the subarachnoid space or the lateral ventricle; or (5) by direct extension of the disease from the middle ear space or from the petrous bone.

Diffuse purulent meningitis is preceded by serous meningitis in the prodromal stage. The onset may be gradual or fulminating. The earliest sign is moderate elevation of temperature accompanied by slight transient headache, which is easily controlled by simple analgesics. The patient may be anxious but is otherwise mentally normal, the tongue is dry and heavily furred and constipation may be marked. Extensor spasm is frequently found, most markedly in the toes. As the disease becomes established, headache is severe and spasmodic, the temperature climbs and the patient becomes confused and irritable. Later, neck stiffness and rigidity occur and the patient is unable to extend his knee when the thigh is flexed on the abdomen – this is Kernig's sign.

In severe meningitis the patient lies curled up on the side, but with the neck extended, frequently with the face buried owing to photophobia, and he or she resents being moved or touched.

Meningitis may complicate acute otitis media or follow a chronic infection of many years' duration. Temperature characteristically climbs, without the periodic fall that occurs in sigmoid sinus thrombosis. The pulse rate shows a steady increase, and blood examination reveals a leucocytosis. Increasing papilloedema may be found on examination of the optic discs, but this is usually a late change. In the final stages hyperpyrexia leads to increasing confusion, coma and death.

Cerebrospinal fluid must be withdrawn by lumbar puncture, and its examination is the most valuable guide to diagnosis. Owing to an increase in cells in meningitis, the fluid becomes turbid and later purulent. Glucose is diminished or absent, protein is increased and pressure rises in the early stages, provided there is free circulation of CSF. There may be many variations from these conditions and the findings must be interpreted as part of the clinical picture. Organisms are now cultured from the CSF in only a minority of cases of meningitis. Most patients have already received antibiotics, so that, although conclusive, the presence of organisms is not necessary for the diagnosis. A swab from the ear may be a useful guide to the organism and its sensitivity, and although by no means all cases of meningitis are otogenic, examination of the ear, nose and sinuses should never be overlooked in a patient with this illness, especially in pneumococcal meningitis.

Differential diagnoses include the various forms of meningitis – tuberculous, meningococcal and pneumococcal; the distinction is made chiefly by CSF examination.

The prognosis depends to some extent on coexistent complications, but with early diagnosis and treatment the outlook is good. Notwithstanding, meningitis is potentially fatal and must be treated promptly. The treatment of meningitis must take priority over the treatment of mastoiditis, but as soon as the patient is sufficiently recovered, surgical treatment of the primary focus can be undertaken as necessary. Mastoidectomy may sometimes be performed earlier in those patients in whom the meningitis is not responding to treatment, but careful consideration must always be given to the possibility that the lack of response is in fact a result of a separate intracranial complication such as an abscess.

Treatment is with broad-spectrum antibiotics given intravenously in full doses. The choice of antibiotic may be altered when the organisms have been isolated and cultured for sensitivity. Intrathecal medication is rarely necessary. If it is used it is vital to administer the type of preparation and dose appropriate to this route of administration. It must be emphasised that lack of response to treatment often indicates a coexistent complication rather than the presence of resistant organisms.

Petrositis

Although not strictly an intracranial complication, petrositis can conveniently be included here. It is the result of extension of infection into the body and apex of the petrous bone.

Petrositis may complicate an acute or chronic otitis media and so occurs in the acute or chronic form of an osteitis or invasion by cholesteatoma. It also occurs as an early or late complication of mastoid operation, during which there may have been interference with aeration or drainage of the petrous cells. Infection reaches the petrous cells by various routes.

The main symptom is headache, which is characteristically spasmodic and felt deep behind the eye. There may be an abducent (VIth) nerve palsy,

caused by oedema affecting the canal in which the nerve runs below the petroclinoid ligament at the apex of the petrous bone. The triad of otorrhoea, retro-orbital pain and abducent nerve palsy is known as Gradenigo's syndrome.

If there has been no previous surgical treatment, the mastoid operation appropriate to the mastoid disease is performed; that is, a cortical or radical mastoidectomy. In either operation careful search is made for any track leading medially into the petrous bone and, if found, this is opened up. With free drainage and intense antibiotic therapy the petrous bone has strong powers of recovery.

Elaborate surgical procedures to open the petrous apex are sometimes needed in rare cases of cholesteatomatous invasion. In these patients it is necessary to use one of several well-described approaches to the petrous bone. Some involve mobilisation and rerouting of the facial nerve; others the removal of the inner ear. Only in this way can all the disease be cleared. Total clearance is sometimes impossible, however, and the surgeon must accept that exteriorisation of disease may be the only practical option.

OPERATIONS FOR MASTOIDITIS AND ITS COMPLICATIONS

Full descriptions of major ear operations are beyond the scope of this book; the reader should, however, have a general understanding of what is involved. What follows are brief descriptions of standard methods of performing this type of surgery; many variations exist, especially in terms of surgical approach.

Cortical mastoidectomy for acute mastoiditis

The patient is prepared and consent for surgery obtained in the usual manner. Although generally performed under general anaesthesia administered via an endotracheal tube (the laryngeal mask airway is not recommended), the procedure can be undertaken under local anaesthesia with sedation. The patient lies supine with the head turned to the side. A postauricular incision is made 1 cm behind the skinfold, following the curve of the auricle. The soft tissues are elevated from the periosteum and retractors are inserted to expose the mastoid cortex.

Cortical bone is removed over a wide area, from Macewan's triangle anterosuperiorly to the mastoid tip inferiorly and the sigmoid sinus region posteriorly. When the cortex is opened, pus may flow and a large cavity may be found filled with necrotic debris, granulation tissue and pus. Further cortical bone is removed widely (Fig. 5.2). The antrum is located, all diseased bone removed and all diseased cells opened.

There are several potential difficulties with this procedure. It should be self-evident that a thorough knowledge of the surgical anatomy of the temporal bone is required, as important structures such as the facial nerve and horizontal semicircular canal may easily be damaged. In a sclerotic acellular mastoid, locating the antrum may be difficult. The sigmoid sinus or dura may be injured.

posterior canal wall

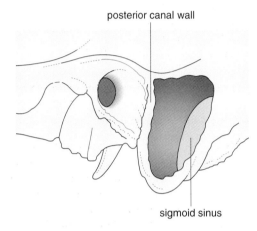

sigmoid sinus

Fig. 5.2 Cortical mastoidectomy (also called a 'simple mastoidectomy'). The posterior canal wall remains intact. The sigmoid sinus is shown; normally a thin plate of bone is left over this, although it may have been eroded by disease. The cavity communicates with the middle ear cleft via the antrum.

> **Key points**
> ➤ The complications of otitis media are potentially life threatening.
> ➤ 'Masked' mastoiditis is more commonly seen than acute mastoiditis in countries where antibiotics are widely available.
> ➤ An intracranial complication may be the presenting feature of chronic suppurative otitis media.

Inner ear

6

SENSORINEURAL HEARING LOSS

Sensorineural hearing loss refers to impairment resulting from abnormalities in the cochlea, auditory nerve, brainstem or higher auditory centres. The distinction between 'sensory' and 'neural' hearing loss has been discussed in Chapter 2. Other equivalent labels that have been used include 'cochlear' and 'retrocochlear' hearing loss.

The obvious symptom of sensorineural hearing loss is deafness but there may be other symptoms of inner ear or auditory pathway dysfunction, such as tinnitus (see below) and vertigo. As well as simple hearing loss, patients may complain of distortion of hearing, unusual difficulty in hearing when there is background noise, or impaired discrimination ('I can hear people but I can't make out what they say'). They may experience difficulty in localising sound or have an abnormal intolerance of even quite mild levels of noise.

Symptoms become more severe as involvement affects more of the speech range of frequencies. High frequencies are usually affected first, and hence the consonants that are so important for the discrimination of speech sounds.

The tympanic membrane is usually normal and air conduction is better than bone conduction on tuning fork tests. The usual audiometric pattern is a sloping loss, the hearing being worse in the high frequencies, but other patterns may occur.

Presbyacusis

With advancing age it is normal for hearing to deteriorate; this is termed 'presbyacusis'. It is not a disease, rather it is a term acknowledging the association between ageing and hearing loss. Several different 'types' of presbyacusis have been described. This classification is of very limited clinical usefulness and some of the pathological changes on which it is based are also seen in patients with hearing loss from other causes.

Sudden sensorineural hearing loss

Sensorineural hearing loss may occur suddenly, with or without trauma. The traumatic causes will be considered first.

Ear surgery

Sensorineural deafness may arise following any ear operation and the patient should be warned of this preoperatively. In many instances the risk is extremely small. The risk in stapedectomy (p. 47) has been discussed but all forms of middle ear and mastoid surgery carry a small risk.

Head injury

The trauma of head injury can affect the inner ear in several ways. Temporal bone fractures are not common; they are discussed in Chapter 4. Sensorineural deafness is more common in the case of a transverse fracture. While a major head injury is required to produce labyrinthine concussion, even a relatively moderate blow may produce sensorineural deafness.

Blast injury

An explosive blast may produce injury both as a result of the high intensity of noise and the shock wave. While the most common finding is perforation of the tympanic membranes, sensorineural deafness and tinnitus also occur. In most cases the hearing loss rapidly resolves, but high frequency losses may persist.

Barotrauma

Otitic barotrauma is discussed in Chapter 4. It is sufficient here to highlight the possibility of a perilymph fistula (below) arising in this disorder. Note also that inner ear decompression sickness is another possible cause of audiovestibular dysfunction following diving.

Perilymph fistula

A perilymph fistula is an abnormal communication between the perilymphatic space and the middle ear – most commonly it occurs through a defect in the round window membrane or via a breach in the ligament between the stapes footplate and the oval window. In addition to sudden sensorineural hearing loss, the leak is usually associated with vestibular symptoms.

There is little doubt that a fistula can arise as a result of trauma, including direct trauma to the ossicular chain. Postoperative fistulae may also occur. In these cases, exploration of the middle ear and the plugging of any soft tissue defect are appropriate.

Controversy surrounds the concept that a fistula might be produced by more minor trauma, for example barotrauma or the trauma associated with physical exertions such as straining, lifting, coughing, laughing, vomiting, etc. More controversial still is the notion that a 'spontaneous' perilymph fistula may be a cause of sudden sensorineural deafness.

If there is a clear history of a sudden onset of sensorineural deafness and vertigo occurring at the time of an episode of exertion, it seems reasonable to consider this diagnosis. When the diagnosis is in doubt, a period of conservative treatment is warranted. Bed-rest with the head raised is advised. Many cases will settle spontaneously. If symptoms progress or fail to improve, the ear should be surgically explored.

Sudden sensorineural deafness without trauma (idiopathic sudden sensorineural hearing loss)

Sudden sensorineural deafness in the absence of trauma is a medical emergency. In some cases the cause is immediately apparent: occasionally those disorders that are usually associated with deafness of gradual onset present in this way. Sudden deafness may sometimes accompany 'giddiness' (below). Notwithstanding, in a sizeable majority no cause is found and the condition is then termed 'idiopathic sudden sensorineural hearing loss'. This is a diagnosis of exclusion; a thorough search should be made for an identifiable cause. It must be remembered that the attack may mark an initial episode of Ménière's disease or, rarely but importantly, be the presenting feature of an acoustic neuroma.

Spontaneous recovery of hearing occurs in about a third of patients; a third experience partial recovery; and a third have none. A severe loss, a downward sloping audiogram, high frequency loss and the presence of vertigo are unfavourable prognostic features. While investigations are undertaken to exclude the disorders above, empirical treatment is usually initiated. Many different regimens have been proposed and there is no firm evidence to support the effectiveness of any of them. Those 'treatments' with the most widespread support include:

- a short course of oral steroids (e.g. enteric-coated prednisolone 60 mg/day for 3 days, then 45 mg/day for 3 days, then 30 mg/day for 3 days, then 15 mg/day for 3 days, then stop)
- regular inhalation of carbogen (95% oxygen: 5% carbon dioxide)

● betahistine hydrochloride 16 mg three times a day.

If the differential white cell count suggests a possible viral aetiology the addition of an antiviral agent such as acyclovir should be considered. Bed-rest is often recommended.

Progressive sensorineural hearing loss

Ototoxic drugs

Ototoxic drugs are those that are toxic to the auditory and/or vestibular portions of the inner ear. The most common groups of drugs are shown in Box 6.1.

The aminoglycoside group includes some very useful antibiotics, such as gentamicin. Because their toxic effects are well known, their use always involves a balance between these and their beneficial effects. Great effort must be made to minimise the risk of ototoxicity by keeping plasma levels in a safe range.

If there is a hole in the eardrum, the possibility of hearing loss resulting from the use of aminoglycoside antibiotic-containing eardrops has caused concern. There is, however, very little evidence that this actually occurs. When the middle ear is infected and the mucosa is swollen and oedematous, the medication may have difficulty diffusing into the inner ear. In such patients the risk of developing inner ear dysfunction as a result of not treating an infective process is probably greater than that of the aminoglycoside drops. A short course of drops, the duration titrated against the response to treatment, would seem appropriate. In some parts of the world a topical form of ciprofloxacin (a non-ototoxic medication) is available for use in the ear, making these concerns unnecessary.

■ Box 6.1

Drugs commonly affecting the inner ear

- ■ Aminoglycoside antibiotics
- ■ Quinine and related compounds
- ■ Salicylates
- ■ Loop diuretics

The deafness and tinnitus produced by quinine and related compounds are usually temporary but may be permanent. On the other hand, these symptoms are also produced by the salicylate group, including aspirin (acetylsalicylic acid), and are reversible.

The loop diuretics include frusemide and ethacrynic acid. They may produce permanent or temporary hearing loss but more commonly the latter.

Noise

Noise may damage hearing in two ways. Repeated exposure to continuous noise produces noise-induced hearing loss (NIHL). A sudden burst or impulse of high acoustic energy results in a particular type of NIHL referred to as acoustic trauma.

When evaluating any patient with sensorineural deafness a history of noise exposure is important. Industrial noise exposure (as observed in boilermakers, shipbuilders, steelworkers, etc.) is usually bilateral; hearing loss caused by gunfire occurs in the ear nearest the barrel. Damage results from levels of 85 dB for 8 hours per day and there are now strict guidelines produced by health and safety authorities to protect those who work in noisy environments. Appropriately fitted and worn ear protectors can attenuate sound by up to 30 dB. The hearing loss produced by noise is greatest in the 3–4 kHz region, producing a characteristic notch on the audiogram. When patients with NIHL are seen they should be counselled carefully about the dangers of further exposure to noise.

Autoimmune deafness

The concept of 'autoimmune inner ear disease' is still not widely accepted. The term covers a variety of clinical syndromes in which cell-mediated or humoral-mediated mechanisms produce inner ear dysfunction. Two distinct types are recognised: organ-specific and non-organ-specific. In the former it is postulated that autoantibodies or cell-mediated immune responses against inner ear antigens are present and produce inner ear disease. Rapidly progressive bilateral sensorineural deafness has been attributed to such a process. In non-organ-specific disease a similar clinical picture is observed but only in patients with a coexisting systemic immune disease.

It is important to recognise cases of possible autoimmune inner ear disease because those patients with disabling symptoms may be treated with immunosuppressive medication.

Infections

Labyrinthitis can arise as a complication of otitis media as either infection or toxins spread into the labyrinth. Vertigo may be present in addition to hearing loss, although these features may recover partially or completely as the infection settles. Meningitis may produce sensorineural deafness and is one of the most common causes of severe or profound acquired deafness in infants and children. The deafness is usually bilateral. All patients who have suffered from meningitis, especially children, should have their hearing tested as soon as possible after recovery.

Syphilis is an extremely rare cause of hearing loss but cases do occur. The diagnosis should be considered in patients with unexplained deafness or vertigo, and the appropriate blood tests performed.

Several viruses cause deafness, which is probably why a viral infection is implicated in many cases of acute deafness. There is often an association between sudden deafness and upper respiratory symptoms or an influenzal type of illness, but association does not always imply causation. The effects of some viruses have been clearly defined; the deafness that may occur in herpes zoster oticus (Ramsay Hunt syndrome), for example, will be mentioned later (Ch. 8). Measles and mumps may produce deafness: in mumps the loss is almost always unilateral. Many other viruses have been implicated as a cause of deafness and there is a high prevalence of otological symptoms, including sensorineural hearing loss, in patients with human immunodeficiency virus (HIV) infection and acquired immune deficiency syndrome (AIDS).

Chronic otitis media

There is a greater incidence of high frequency sensorineural hearing loss in patients with chronic otitis media when compared to normal. When a cholesteatoma is present it may erode the bone of the otic capsule, producing a fistula and subsequent loss of auditory and/or vestibular function.

Otosclerosis

Otosclerosis is discussed in detail in Chapter 4. There is controversy about sensorineural hearing loss in patients with otosclerosis. Some believe that toxins damage the inner ear, whereas others assert that the sensorineural loss observed is no greater than one would expect in non-otosclerosis patients of similar age and history. Equally controversial is the idea that otosclerosis can affect the inner ear without signs and symptoms of stapes fixation, producing 'cochlear otosclerosis'.

Sensorineural hearing loss in children

The early identification of children with hearing loss is extremely important. This is particularly the case when a child has a severe or profound sensorineural loss, as early auditory rehabilitation offers the best hope for normal development and education.

Certain groups of children have a high incidence of sensorineural deafness and these should be screened as soon as practicable and, if necessary, at regular intervals thereafter until it is certain that their hearing has been accurately assessed. At risk groups include:

- Those with a family history of deafness, or hereditary defects.
- Infants exposed to prenatal risk factors such as maternal infection (e.g. rubella, syphilis), drug usage, rhesus incompatibility.
- Those with perinatal damage, e.g. anoxia, low birth weight, jaundice.
- Those with specific illnesses in the postnatal period, e.g. measles, mumps, meningitis.

If a child cannot hear properly, then speech cannot develop normally; therefore, if speech development is delayed or abnormal, it is important to test the hearing at an early stage. A child acquires speech by imitation, and the child can only reproduce what he or she hears. At the age of 12 months a child should normally be able to localise familiar sounds. By the age of 2 he or she should understand simple commands and be able to put words together.

If a child's parent is suspicious of a hearing problem a careful assessment must be made; parents are often right.

When examining the hearing-impaired child it is essential to recognise and exclude middle ear problems such as otitis media with effusion (OME), and treat where necessary. If OME is present, a relatively mild loss becomes severe until the middle ear problem is treated. It is equally important that the child with sensorineural deafness is examined to exclude other difficulties of a physical, psychological or behavioural nature. Poor educational achievement and bad behaviour are not always attributable to a hearing problem.

In many children with sensorineural hearing loss there is no obvious cause. In some, deafness occurs as part of a recognisable syndrome or following exposure to one of the risk factors above. The best results for auditory rehabilitation are obtained if the loss is recognised in the first year of life. In children with severe hearing loss, hearing aids must be fitted and special training of residual hearing begun, as soon as the diagnosis is made. With the high quality aids that are now available, an increasing number of these children learn satisfactory speech and a high proportion can be integrated into normal schools. Some children with severe or profound deafness may benefit from cochlear implants (Ch. 7).

The key issues in a child with sensorineural deafness are early diagnosis combined with appropriate rehabilitation.

'GIDDINESS'

Many patients suffer from 'giddiness' and it has been pointed out that even the most enthusiastic doctor may experience a decline in spirits when faced with such patients. Only some of these patients have vertigo; many have a general sense of imbalance, light-headedness, a feeling of falling or some similar symptom, rather than the illusory sense that they or their surroundings are moving (usually spinning), which is characteristic of true vertigo. Vertigo is often associated with systemic disturbances of sweating, nausea or vomiting.

Normal balance is maintained by the complex coordination of input from the visual, vestibular and proprioceptive systems, which are integrated and modulated in the brainstem under the influence of higher cortical centres. The output of this system to the oculomotor and musculoskeletal systems effects the necessary changes in eye and body position. Balance may be disturbed (and 'dizziness' ensue) if there are problems with any part of this system.

The causes of 'dizziness' are shown in Box 6.2. A detailed history is vital if a diagnosis is to be reached. If at the end of the history a specific diagnosis has not been reached, one is rarely forthcoming with extensive examination and tests.

The general medical problems mentioned in Box 6.2 may be evident from the history. The dizziness in these cases is not similar to vertigo and usually consists of light-headedness. The multifactorial nature of balance problems in the elderly can lead to a rather confusing history; note should be taken of any features suggestive of visual, proprioceptive or musculoskeletal disease.

Other signs of ear disease, such as hearing loss and tinnitus, often accompany vertigo of otological origin. Aural discharge may suggest middle ear disease. If the cause of the vertigo lies centrally, one expects to find other symptoms of CNS dysfunction.

The onset and duration of dizziness are important and it is worthwhile focusing quite specifically on the details of the first attack: precipitating factors should be determined — in many cases the patient awakes and is suddenly 'hit' by the vertigo. A short-lived attack (seconds in duration) is usual in benign positional paroxysmal vertigo (BPPV), while Menière's attacks are longer (below). An episode of acute labyrinthine dysfunction usually involves vertigo that continues unabated for many hours. This

Inner ear

■ Box 6.2

Causes of 'dizziness'

Otological
– With hearing loss   Ménière's disease
                        Infective labyrinthitis –
                          including herpes zoster,
                          bacterial, syphilis
                        Trauma – head injury,
                          surgery
                        Perilymph fistula
                        Drugs

– Without   Acute vestibular
  hearing loss   dysfunction
                        Chronic vestibular
                          hypofunction with
                          incomplete
                          compensation or
                          episodic
                          decompensation
                        'Vestibular neuronitis'
                        Drugs
                        Benign positional
                          paroxysmal vertigo
                          (BPPV)

Non-otological
– Neurological   Central (brainstem)
                          vascular disease
                        Demyelination
                        Familial vertigo, ataxia
                          and nystagmus
                        Migraine
                        Posterior fossa tumours

– General   Peripheral vascular disease
                        Hypotensive
                          conditions (postural
                          hypotension, bradycardia,
                          etc.)
                        Diabetes
                        Drugs

situation must be distinguished from that in which a briefer episode of vertigo is followed by a general sense of imbalance.

The eardrums should be examined and the tuning fork tests performed. A systematic examination of the cranial nerves is undertaken. Specifically this should look for the presence of nystagmus and abnormalities of the smooth pursuit mechanism. Ophthalmoscopy allows the fundi to be examined for signs of raised intracranial pressure, small degrees of nystagmus or other subtle eye movement problems. Cerebellar screening tests (such as finger–nose pointing) and simple tests of balance and gait (Romberg's test and Unterberger's stepping test) should be done routinely. Positional testing may be indicated.

Special investigations will follow in selected cases. Audiometry is important in determining the type and extent of hearing loss. Electronystagmography allows spontaneous nystagmus to be recorded with and without fixation, optokinetic nystagmus can be assessed and smooth pursuit examined. Caloric testing allows each labyrinth to be stimulated independently to assess symmetry of vestibular inputs. More advanced tests of vestibular function include rotatory chair and dynamic platform testing. In addition to these tests of vestibular function, the auditory nerve, brainstem and cerebral structure can be evaluated with CT and MRI.

Even in cases in which all these investigations have been undertaken, there remains a proportion of patients in whom the diagnosis is uncertain; however, patients with true rotatory vertigo and no central signs of symptoms will probably have a peripheral vestibular disorder. Further management depends on the nature of the dysfunction.

Acute unilateral vestibular failure or impairment

This will result in vertigo of sudden onset. The symptoms will continue until the vestibular input to higher centres becomes 'symmetrical' again. This will occur when either (1) the dysfunction has resolved and both vestibules send equal input to the brainstem; or (2) despite continuing unequal input from the periphery, the vestibular nuclei in the brainstem produce equal output for higher centres. This last process is known as central compensation.

The process of compensation is shown in Figure 6.1. Many patients who have in the past been diagnosed as having 'labyrinthitis' or 'vestibular neuronitis' (below) are now probably more appropriately thought of as having an episode of 'acute vestibular dysfunction'. The former terms imply that a specific pathophysiological process might have taken place, but this is often conjectural. Infection *may* spread to the labyrinth, as a consequence of acute or chronic otitis media, producing labyrinthitis. An 'epidemic' of vertigo may suggest that a viral agent is responsible; in many cases the nature of the precipitating event is irrelevant.

Several key management points should be noted. Firstly, vestibular sedatives such as prochlorperazine have a role in aborting vertiginous sensations in the early acute phase of a prolonged attack of vertigo. Their continued use cannot, however, be recommended. They may delay compensation and reduce still further the remaining vestibular function in patients who can ill afford such a reduction. Secondly, immobility can also delay compensation. For many years exercise regimens (such as the Cooksey–Cawthorne exercises) have been available and these are designed to stress the balance system in a safe and regulated environment. More recently these have been replaced by vestibular therapy programmes, tailored to individual patients' needs. Young people can expect to achieve complete compensation, but this process can be delayed, even incomplete, in the elderly. Incomplete compensation results in difficulty in coping with situations in which the balance system is stressed. In the young this may only rarely occur – for example, when turning quickly; elderly patients, however, often have compromise of the other sensory modalities contributing to normal balance-vision and proprioception. It would be surprising if the patient with poor vision (cataracts, for example), poor proprioception (arthritis of several joints, perhaps even a prosthetic joint or two) and poor, uncompensated vestibular function did *not* have balance problems. These patients need aids to stability such as sticks and frames as well as to vision: they may also benefit from focused vestibular therapy. They will not be helped by long-term vestibular sedatives, and the temptation to prescribe these should be avoided.

Menière's disease

Menière's syndrome is characterised by recurrent episodes of spontaneous vertigo, fluctuating hearing loss, tinnitus and a feeling of fullness in the ear. There is sometimes an obvious cause for the syndrome (post-traumatic, postinfectious, syphilitic, classic Cogan's syndrome or atypical Cogan's syndrome) but it is usually idiopathic and this is Menière's disease.

The term 'endolymphatic hydrops' is sometimes used interchangeably with Menière's disease or syndrome, as the theory that hydrops is responsible for Menière's syndrome is dominant in current thinking. This remains unproven and hydrops may be an epiphenomenon simply indicating inner ear

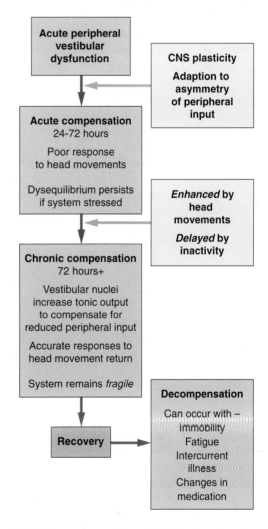

Fig. 6.1 The processes of compensation and decompensation following acute vestibular dysfunction.

dysfunction. An increase in endolymphatic pressure is postulated as the cause for ballooning of Reissner's membrane into the scala vestibuli. The saccular wall balloons outwards to contact the opposite wall of the vestibule, including, eventually, the footplate. With advanced disease, sensory hair cells are lost.

The increased pressure in the endolymph is said to be responsible for the feeling of fullness in the ear, the distortion of hearing, loudness recruitment and dysequilibrium. The ruptures are responsible for acute episodes of vertigo. It is likely that Menière's syndrome is multifactorial in origin and hereditary elements may combine with a wide variety of external stimuli.

The symptoms of Menière's disease usually start in middle age. Men and women are equally affected, although women present more often. The 'classic' Menière's attack consists of a feeling of fullness in the ear accompanied by increasing tinnitus, reduced hearing and the sudden onset of rotatory vertigo. This may last from 20 minutes to several hours and be accompanied by autonomic symptoms such as nausea, vomiting and sweating; the patient does not lose consciousness. The attack can come on at any time, even during sleep. After the acute vertigo has stopped, the patient continues to feel unwell and the balance is poor, often for the rest of the day.

Between attacks it is not uncommon for the patient to experience fullness in the ear, tinnitus or positional vertigo, or simply instability with quick movements. Alternatively the patient may be completely asymptomatic. There is great variability in the pattern of the disease. Some patients have only one or two attacks per year and their hearing is relatively stable. Others have periods of frequent attacks for weeks or months, then periods of remission. Some are totally incapacitated by their disease.

The audiogram shows a low tone loss. Loudness recruitment is present so the patient may develop hyperacusis and be intolerant of loud noises.

Diagnostic difficulties occur when the full set of symptoms is not present. The syndrome may begin with hearing loss, vertigo or tinnitus alone, although the latter two presentations are unusual.

The history is the most important factor in making the diagnosis of Menière's disease. Several diagnostic tests have been advocated, in particular electrocochleography. Unfortunately the poor test/retest reliability and the low sensitivity and specificity of this test make its usefulness questionable. It is of dubious value in establishing or refuting the diagnosis in patients with equivocal histories.

Medical treatment of Menière's disease aims to reduce the number and severity of attacks and minimise the symptoms during an individual attack. The patient is encouraged to follow a low salt diet, as this is believed to reduce inner ear pressure. Betahistine hydrochloride is prescribed, and a mild diuretic can also be added. Acute attacks may be aborted by the use of a vestibular sedative such as prochlorperazine; sublabial versions are available to avoid the problems of swallowing while feeling nauseous.

More invasive therapies may be considered if medical treatment fails to control the patient's symptoms. Menière's disease has a high natural resolution rate and several placebo-controlled studies have shown some placebos to be remarkably effective in controlling symptoms. It has even been suggested that simply contemplating surgery may lead to a clinical improvement.

Surgery for Menière's disease may aim to preserve hearing while reducing or abolishing vestibular function, or it may be destructive, destroying both hearing and balance in the affected ear. Endolymphatic sac decompression is one of the least invasive surgical procedures. A cortical mastoidectomy is performed and the sac identified and incised, and a drain inserted. The procedure does not usually affect hearing. Vestibular nerve section, on the other hand, is more invasive. The nerve can be sectioned (preserving the cochlear nerve and hearing), via a retrolabyrinthine approach or via the middle cranial fossa, to eliminate the vertiginous symptoms. There is a risk of hearing loss and facial palsy with this procedure.

If hearing is poor and unserviceable a formal labyrinthectomy may be performed, destroying the inner ear. This can be undertaken through the middle ear or via a mastoidectomy approach. All hearing is lost. Recently, medical labyrinthectomy with hearing preservation using intratympanic gentamicin has become popular.

Benign positional paroxysmal vertigo (BPPV)

In this disorder vertigo occurs when the head is in a particular position. It may follow a head injury but a precipitating cause is not usually evident. The symptoms result from a lesion of the crista of the posterior semicircular canal. It is believed that one of the otolith crystals becomes displaced, finding its way into the canal. When the patient rotates the head (often while turning in bed) an abnormally strong signal from the affected canal produces transient rotatory vertigo. There is no hearing loss, and the symptoms usually abate spontaneously after 3–6 months. There are characteristic signs on positional testing (Ch. 2); these are a short latent interval, followed by rotatory, geotropic nystagmus. The nystagmus adapts and fatigues. If this does not happen, central positional nystagmus should be suspected and further investigations initiated.

Medication is of no value. Treatment has been revolutionised by the canalith repositioning manoeuvres such as the Epley manoeuvre (Fig. 6.2).

Labyrinthitis

Labyrinthitis can develop when bacteria, or the toxins they produce, enter the labyrinth. This condition has been discussed as a complication of otitis media. Vertigo is associated with sensorineural hearing loss. Many patients with 'giddiness' are said to have labyrinthitis but this is extremely unlikely, it is often more accurate to say that they have an episode of acute vestibular (and sometimes cochlear) dysfunction, and not presume that intralabyrinthine inflammation is the cause.

Vestibular neuronitis

Vestibular neuronitis is a diagnosis usually made in otherwise healthy patients who experience a sudden attack of vertigo. An apparent association with upper respiratory viral infections and the suggestion that 'epidemics' of the disorder occur within communities have led to the idea that a viral infection of the vestibular ganglion is responsible. There is almost no histological evidence that this is the case. The symptoms and signs are those of acute vestibular failure, cochlear involvement being notably absent. Treatment is symptomatic while waiting for recovery to occur by compensation.

Lateral medullary syndrome

Severe paroxysmal vertigo with vomiting occurs with other neurological signs of medullary infarction. These include ipsilateral paraesthesia and paralysis of the soft palate, larynx and pharynx, and contralateral paraesthesia of the limbs and trunk. Hearing loss may occur.

Drug toxicity

The effect of certain drugs on the inner ear has already been mentioned. A non-specific effect on the vestibular system can arise from a wide variety of drugs, but generally well-defined dizziness does not occur. Drugs that are usually to blame are those given for epilepsy (especially phenytoin), those used in depression and anxiety, and some antihypertensive agents (especially ganglion blockers).

Vertebrobasilar ischaemia

Episodes of dysequilibrium often arise in patients with vascular disease. The diagnosis of vertebrobasilar insufficiency should, however, only be made when there are other neurological signs of transient ischaemia: these might include amaurosis fugax, drop attacks, weakness of the extremities or slurred speech. A cervical collar may be useful if symptoms are aggravated by turning the head.

NEUROLOGICAL DISORDERS

Vestibular schwannoma (acoustic neuroma)

In the past the most common tumour of the cochleovestibular nerve was known as an 'acoustic neuroma'. This is a misnomer because the tumour

Inner ear

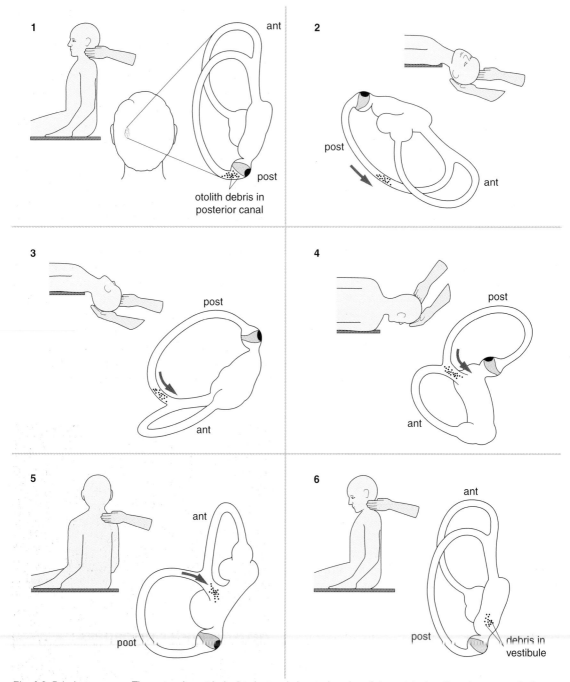

Fig. 6.2 Epley's manoeuvre. The patient lies with the head extended over the edge of the couch, the affected ear towards the floor. (2) The head is rotated through 90° towards the opposite ear (3) and then through a further 90° until the face points towards the floor (4) Finally the patient is brought into a sitting position with the chin down (5 & 6).

arises from the Schwann cells covering the superior or inferior vestibular nerves, and the preferred name is vestibular schwannoma. These tumours account for 6–10% of all intracranial tumours and 80–90% of all tumours in the cerebellopontine angle. They arise in the internal auditory canal at the glial–Schwann cell junction. They are slow-growing, benign tumours which do not infiltrate local tissues or metastasise. However, as they grow they compress adjacent tissues and, in common with other benign intracranial tumours, the effects of this pressure may be extremely serious. Within the internal auditory canal the tumours only affect the vestibular and cochlear nerves (the facial nerve is extremely resistant to pressure) but when the tumour starts to grow out of the internal canal it pushes medially, superiorly and inferiorly. Pressure on the brainstem may eventually produce a rise in intracranial pressure and death may ensue.

The cause of most vestibular schwannomas is unknown. Neurofibromatosis types 1 (NF1) and 2 (NF2) are associated with vestibular schwannomas. Bilateral vestibular schwannomas are common in NF2 but the incidence of these tumours in NF1 is low. In non-neurofibromatosis cases men and women are affected equally and the mean age at diagnosis is about 50. Progressive unilateral sensorineural deafness is the most common clinical presentation; however, the hearing loss may be sudden in 15–25% of cases. Other features include unilateral or asymmetric tinnitus (occasionally the only symptom) or balance disturbance. The latter is not often a prominent feature because the slow growth of the tumour allows central compensation to occur. If the tumour becomes large, more sinister symptoms may develop. These include cerebellar symptoms of motor incoordination, pain or paraesthesia in the face as a result of involvement of the trigeminal (Vth cranial) nerve, or finally headaches, diplopia and vomiting caused by raised intracranial pressure.

The audiogram shows asymmetrical sensorineural hearing loss, usually worse in the higher frequencies. Speech discrimination is reduced to a greater degree than would be expected from the audiogram. Occasionally the audiogram appears normal.

The diagnostic test of choice is MRI (Fig. 6.3). The test is non-invasive and free of the risks of exposure to X-rays. CT may detect large tumours and those arising in the internal canal that have widened it. With CT, small intracanalicular tumours will be missed. In the past a range of audiovestibular tests have been used as screening tools to select those patients in whom MRI might be most appropriate. These include brainstem evoked response audiometry and caloric testing (q.v.). There is always a significant false-positive and false-negative rate with these tests and, if at all possible, MRI is preferred.

Management of a patient with a vestibular schwannoma depends on several factors, most importantly the size of the tumour and the patient's general medical condition. In patients whose medical condition and/or age make the risks of surgery greater than usual, it may be appropriate to monitor the growth of the tumour with regular scans and defer treatment, perhaps indefinitely. The argument against this 'watchful waiting' approach is that

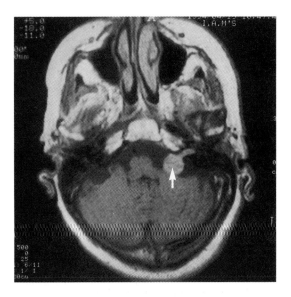

Fig. 6.3 MRI scan showing acoustic neuroma.

Inner ear

surgical risk is likely to increase as the tumour grows and the patient gets older, and fitness diminishes. Radiosurgery treatment is another non-surgical option, but the merits or otherwise of this treatment modality are still not clear.

The aim of surgical treatment is to remove the tumour and prevent the risks associated with continued tumour growth. If the patient has serviceable hearing a secondary aim may be preservation of hearing. Whenever possible, facial nerve function should be preserved but its proximity to the tumour puts it at risk during surgery.

Several different surgical approaches are available. In the translabyrinthine approach the internal auditory canal is reached via the mastoid by removing the bony labyrinth: hearing is inevitably destroyed. The retrosigmoid approach is a more invasive procedure involving opening the skull with a craniotomy and retraction of the cerebellum – there may be long-term sequelae. The internal canal can be approached from above via the middle cranial fossa.

TINNITUS

The patient with tinnitus experiences sounds that *appear* to originate in the head. There are various real sounds that *are* created in the head, in both normal and abnormal conditions. These are not regarded as tinnitus in the normal sense of the word; they have been termed 'somato-sounds'. Such normal sounds arise from the temporomandibular joint, the eustachian tube, the movements of muscles and joints and from the normal blood vessels near the ear. Patients sometimes need reassurance that noises arising from these sources are normal and of no significance. Other noises may arise in abnormal circumstances, for example from vascular tumours in or near the ear, or the increased vascularity arising from an acute infection in the ear. In all these cases the sound is more easily heard in a very quiet room or if there is a conductive hearing loss present, as there is no masking effect from the ordinary outside environment. In 'objective tinnitus' there is a real noise that can be heard by an observer as well as the patient. This is extremely rare but can occur with vascular abnormalities, large vascular tumours and occasionally in

palatal myoclonus, in which a rhythmic clicking of the eustachian tube is heard.

The most common type of tinnitus is that which is associated with sensorineural hearing loss, although such loss may not always be detectable using standard pure-tone audiometry. In these patients, abnormal neuronal activity is thought to be responsible for the auditory percept known as tinnitus. This activity may be wholly or partially generated in the central nervous system, however, rather than peripherally in the cochlea, even when the basic underlying pathology is in the cochlea.

The 'cochlear model' for tinnitus states that it is another manifestation of the cochlear disorder which produces the hearing loss: the brain interprets abnormal rates or rhythms of discharge in the cochlear nerve fibres as tinnitus. Several factors may trigger the onset of this process, including for example stress (emotional, physical or behavioural), ear surgery or syringing, head or whiplash injury or pressure changes.

The model is elaborated by two further components. Firstly, the abnormal neuronal activity leads to an increase in the brain's attention to sound. This is responsible for the increased intrusiveness of tinnitus and the hyperacusis (a decreased tolerance to noise) observed in some patients. Secondly, the anxiety caused by the tinnitus and the patient's attention to it produces tension and further enhances the patient's attentional focus on the tinnitus: its intrusiveness consequently increases and it becomes yet more aggravating. In this way a vicious cycle is established.

Tinnitus usually has a buzzing, hissing or ringing quality. It may be intermittent or continuous, unilateral or bilateral, and stress and tiredness often make it worse. It is usually more noticeable in bed at night when background noise is at its quietest.

A full otological history should be elicited from every tinnitus patient and a thorough examination performed. Any specific cause should be identified, if necessary after the appropriate radiological and serological investigations. Unilateral tinnitus as a potential symptom of an acoustic neuroma has been mentioned above. Hearing tests are extremely important for both diagnostic and rehabilitative purposes.

It is crucial that the patient with tinnitus is managed appropriately from the first point of contact with any healthcare professional. Negative professional counselling and reinforcement of popularly held but erroneous beliefs – 'there's nothing wrong with you, nothing can be done and you'll just have to learn to live with it – are extremely unhelpful. A positive approach focuses on treating those patients with identifiable and remediable pathology and providing appropriate psychological and prosthetic support to all patients. The importance of psychological help cannot be emphasised enough. This includes professional counselling from the doctor (general practitioner and specialist) and hearing therapist or audiologist. Details of such counselling are beyond the scope of this book but include careful explanation of the nature of the tinnitus, specific reassurance that the patient does not have any sinister intracranial disease, that the tinnitus will not damage their hearing and that it is unlikely to continue unabated. The favourable prognosis in the majority of patients must be emphasised. This professional counselling can, and should when possible, be supported by literature. There may be a role for other psychological counselling techniques and for relaxation therapy.

Hearing aids and white noise generators (previously known as 'tinnitus maskers') are the prosthetic devices used in tinnitus retraining therapy and masking. Retraining therapy aims to produce long-term reduction in tinnitus intrusiveness; masking provides a background level of sound against which the loudness of the tinnitus is reduced.

There is a limited but important role for medication with tinnitus patients and this is princi-pally in managing its effects. In some patients the short-term and focused use of antidepressants or tranquillisers and/or sedatives to aid sleep may be appropriate. Surgery has a very limited place in management. It is attractive to imagine that cutting the cochlear nerve will abolish tinnitus in most patients; this is not the case. Several mechanical devices, involving electrical or magnetic stimulation of the cochlea, have been described, but at present none has been shown to be consistently useful.

> **Key points**
> ➤ Sudden sensorineural deafness is a medical emergency.
> ➤ Early diagnosis and appropriate rehabilitation are important in the child with sensorineural deafness.
> ➤ Not all 'dizzy' patients have vertigo.
> ➤ Acute vestibular impairment is usually followed by central compensation.
> ➤ Vestibular sedatives are useful in acute vertigo but long-term use may delay compensation.
> ➤ Menière's disease has specific and characteristic features.
> ➤ Asymmetrical audiovestibular symptoms may be due to a vestibular schwannoma (acoustic neuroma).
> ➤ Initial management of the tinnitus patient is important; negative professional counselling must be avoided.

Aids to hearing

Identifying the type of hearing loss is one of the most important factors in determining the ease with which a patient may be helped. Some patients with a conductive loss may be helped surgically. Alternatively, a hearing aid may be used: even simple aids may be useful because the hearing loss can be overcome by increasing the volume of the presented sound. Since the inner ear functions normally in most patients with conductive losses, provided amplification is adequate the patient hears clearly. For patients with a sensorineural loss, relief by means of a hearing aid is more complex. Not only does an aid have to provide amplification, it has to cope with other aspects of the patient's disability, such as recruitment, a narrow band of loudness discomfort and, perhaps most difficult of all, impairment of speech discrimination (Ch. 2).

HEARING AIDS

Non-electrical

Ear trumpets and speaking tubes still have an occasional use, especially in elderly patients with severe sensorineural hearing loss who have difficulty handling electrical devices. Distortion is minimal and background noise not troublesome but they are very conspicuous.

Electrical

These consist essentially of a microphone, a receiver and an amplifier. They may be body-worn devices (below) but more usually are worn behind the ear (BTE), in the ear (ITE) or in the canal (ITC). In the BTE device sound is led from the aid through a thin transparent plastic tube to a skeleton mould fitted in the concha. Several types of device exist, some relying on new digital technology. Many instruments incorporate a T (telecoil) switch. This allows the microphone on the aid to be disconnected and the instrument driven instead by the signal from a telephone or loop system such as may be found in theatres or lecture halls. In this way background noise is eliminated. The majority of patients, even those with a moderately severe loss, can be fitted with an ear-level device of this type. If hearing loss is bilateral, bilateral aids may be appropriate. ITE and ITC aids offer cosmetic advantages but may not be suitable for all; they are also expensive.

The CROS (contralateral routing of signals) aid brings sound from a microphone behind one ear, via a fine wire, to an insert in the other ear. This can be useful if a patient has no usefully amplifiable hearing on one side but reasonable levels on the other.

For patients with a very severe hearing loss a more powerful instrument is needed and a body-worn device may be necessary. This may be concealed behind clothing but is connected by a wire to a receiver in a moulded acrylic insert which fits in the conchal bowl.

The aids described above are air conduction aids. Bone conduction aids may be necessary in patients with intractable otitis externa, chronically discharging ears or mastoid cavities or meatal stenosis who cannot tolerate the usual insert in the ear. In the past the aid consisted of a vibrator placed on the mastoid bone and held in position by a head band, but now the device can be attached to a percutaneous titanium plug passing through the skin behind the ear into the cortical bone of the skull (Fig. 7.1). This method uses techniques of osseointegration, and results are excellent.

Whatever type of aid is fitted and whatever the type of hearing loss, perseverance and intelligence are needed to make the fullest use of any device. Close cooperation with a hearing therapist is necessary. Training in the use of residual hearing is important and lip reading should be encouraged. It is important that an aid is optimally fitted and of the correct type before a patient judges its suitability. In addition the patient should try using it at home, at work and while undertaking leisure activities. This is particularly important if an aid is purchased privately.

OTHER AIDS TO HEARING

In addition to hearing aids, many other devices and strategies are available to help the hearing impaired. Environmental aids (also known as 'assistive listening devices') are of various types. For patients with severe hearing loss it is a simple matter to fit the main living room with a loop system. This consists of a simple wire encircling the room near floor level. Signals from the television, radio, baby alarm and door bell can be fed into this loop, which generates an electromagnetic field to activate the hearing aid. This system permits freedom of movement

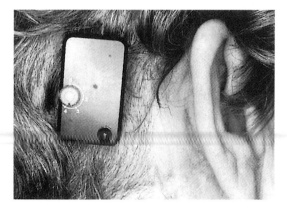

Fig. 7.1 Bone-anchored hearing aid. The aid is attached to a titanium implant which passes through the skin and is anchored in the bone of the skull. The device is sited within the hair line and is unobtrusive.

that an alternative, a direct link to the television for example, does not. This domestic loop system is similar to those available in public places such as theatres and concert halls. An alternative is an invisible infrared light beam that can be used to carry a signal from a television set to a hearing aid.

In several countries television companies provide special services for the hearing impaired. These include the provision of subtitles and of programmes accompanied by a sign-language translator. Buzzers and flashing lights are available to replace normal door or telephone bells and an under-the-pillow vibrator can be used by patients who would not ordinarily hear their alarm clock.

Listening strategies and lip-reading skills can be taught to those with hearing loss. The availability of hearing therapists is increasing and it is hoped that in the future more patients will become familiar with these facilities and able to see them demonstrated.

COCHLEAR IMPLANTS

Cochlear implants have an increasingly important place in the management of adults and children with severe or profound deafness. They are suitable for those with bilateral sensorineural hearing loss who are not able to derive significant benefit from optimally fitted conventional hearing aids. The device consists of two components – internal and external. A small microphone behind the patient's ear picks up sound and sends it via a wire to a speech processor. Traditionally, these were small boxes worn on the belt but newer models look like normal BTE hearing aids and are worn in that way. The processor analyses the signal and the output stimulates a small induction coil held in position on the side of the head by a small magnet. This external component lies over the surgically implanted internal part of the device, which consists of a small receiver–stimulator package that receives its power and information from the external coil. The package produces electrical impulses which pass down a slender multielectrode array, surgically inserted into the basal turn of the cochlea. As various electrodes are stimulated, neural elements of the cochlea are excited and an auditory percept is produced (Fig. 7.2).

The best results are seen in patients who have acquired speech and language before losing their hearing and are implanted as short a time after the onset of deafness as possible. Children who are born with profound sensorineural deafness, or who lose hearing before acquiring speech, may also benefit from the device. In principle, the younger the age at which they are implanted, the greater this benefit because full advantage can then be taken of the inherent 'plasticity' of the auditory central nervous system. Implantation must only be considered, however, when the diagnosis is certain and appropriate aids have been tried.

Awareness of environmental sounds is the minimum achievement one would expect from the user of an implant. The majority of adults find it an aid to lip reading and the best users can communicate on the telephone with the device.

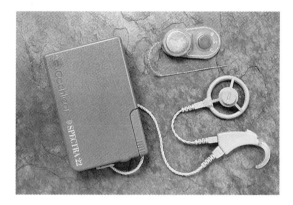

Fig. 7.2 Cochlear implant. The implanted device is shown top right. The thin intracochlear electrode can be seen. Below is the microphone worn behind the ear (bottom right) and attached to it the coil (centre right), which transmits information and power across the skin. The speech processor is shown on the left.

> ► **Key points**
> ► A wide variety of hearing and environmental aids are available.
> ► Patients with conductive hearing loss do particularly well with hearing aids.
> ► Cochlear implants are suitable for some patients with severe or profound sensorineural hearing loss.

Facial nerve

8

CAUSES OF FACIAL PARALYSIS

Facial weakness is usually a result of damage to the lower motor neurone facial nerve fibres somewhere along their course. This can conveniently be divided into three sections:

- intracranial section (from the pons, across the cerebellopontine angle to the meatus of the internal auditory canal
- intratemporal section (internal auditory canal to geniculate ganglion, then horizontal and descending portions)
- extratemporal section (stylomastoid foramen through the parotid to the facial muscles).

Damage to the upper motor neurones is much rarer. It may be recognised by the sparing of the upper facial muscles and preservation of emotional movements.

Paralysis may be partial or complete. The face can be considered in sections – forehead, eye, nose, mouth – and the degree of weakness in each section noted. When the eye rolls upwards during attempted eye closure this is Bell's phenomenon (*not* to be confused with Bell's palsy, below) and is said to indicate a lower motor neurone lesion.

Intracranial lesions are usually tumours in the cerebellopontine angle. If the lesion is large, other neighbouring cranial nerves may be affected, especially the VIIIth (producing hearing loss), Vth and the lower cranial nerves.

Intratemporal lesions may occur as a complication of acute or chronic middle ear disease. In some patients the facial nerve canal in the middle ear is dehiscent, and pus in the middle ear in acute otitis media results in a palsy. Cholesteatoma may erode

the facial canal and this is still occasionally the presenting feature of this condition. Palsy may be a feature of malignant otitis externa (q.v.). It may also occur as a result of trauma, such as a fracture of the temporal bone or operative accident. Other intratemporal causes include herpes zoster oticus and Bell's palsy, which are discussed below.

Extratemporal causes include trauma, either direct or operative, and tumours such as parotid carcinoma.

BELL'S PALSY

The most common type of lower motor neurone facial paralysis is Bell's palsy, accounting for three-quarters of acute facial palsies. It is imperative that this term is used for idiopathic lesions and not as a synonym for 'facial palsy'. Until thorough investigation has excluded other identifiable causes, the term should not be used. As true Bell's palsies usually recover, a facial palsy that does not recover should not be termed a Bell's palsy.

Bell's palsy is usually of rapid onset and evolution and may be associated with pain and numbness of the ear, the midface and the tongue. The patient may also experience a disturbance of taste and associated neuropathies of other cranial nerves. About one-third of patients have only a partial weakness and are likely to make an excellent recovery. In the majority of patients, signs of recovery begin within 4–6 weeks of onset and complete recovery is likely in these patients too. In the remainder, sequelae in the form of persisting weakness and synkinesis occur more frequently.

All patients with Bell's palsy should consult an otolaryngologist and a full ENT examination should be undertaken. An audiogram and tympanometry should be performed to identify any coexistent hearing loss or middle ear disorder. If the palsy does not recover, an MRI scan of the cerebellopontine angle and skull base should be obtained. A variety of 'topodiagnostic' tests have been described to determine the site of a lesion along the course of the nerve; these are unreliable* and of doubtful value.

If a Bell's palsy is complete and the patient is seen soon after the onset of paralysis, he or she may be treated with a short course of steroids, gradually diminishing in dosage. Providing steroids are not contraindicated, a course of enteric coated prednisolone 60 mg/day for 3 days, followed by 45 mg/day for 3 days, 30 mg/day for 3 days and 15 mg/day for a final 3 days, is usually satisfactory. There is some evidence that such treatment is useful in complete palsies but it is insufficient to justify this recommendation in patients with incomplete palsies. It has been suggested that Bell's palsy is a form of viral neuritis and antiviral agents such as acyclovir have been recommended; good evidence of their effectiveness is awaited. Whatever medical treatment is instituted, appropriate eye care is essential. Failure of eye closure may result in a dry, painful eye with corneal damage unless steps are taken to prevent this. If in doubt, involve an ophthalmologist in the patient's care.

HERPES ZOSTER OTICUS

Herpes zoster oticus (Ramsay Hunt syndrome) accounts for less than 10% of acute facial palsies but is an important diagnosis to make. The palsy is produced by a neuritis caused by the herpes zoster virus. The characteristic features are otalgia and varicelliform eruptions in the external ear or soft palate, and the patient may also have hearing loss and vertigo as a result of the involvement of the VIIIth cranial nerve and weakness of nerves V, IX and X. The patient should be treated with appropriate antiviral agents but the prognosis is more guarded than in Bell's palsy, nearly half of the patients experiencing major sequelae.

> **Key points**

> ➤ Not all acute facial palsies are Bell's palsy.
> ➤ A 'Bell's palsy' that does not recover is not a Bell's palsy.
> ➤ Steroids may be of value in patients with complete facial palsies seen early after their onset.

THE NOSE AND PARANASAL SINUSES

2

Anatomy and physiology of the nose and paranasal sinuses

9

STRUCTURE OF THE NOSE

The external nose is supported by bone and cartilage. The bony part is formed mainly by the nasal bones on each side, and the frontal process of the maxillary bone. The cartilaginous portion is formed by several cartilages which support and give shape to the lower part of the nose and nasal tips (Fig. 9.1). Attached to the cartilages are the muscles for dilating the nares.

The nasal cavity has its axis at right angles to the face. It is important to remember this fact when examining the nose, as it is a common misconception that the nasal axis is parallel to the line of the external nasal structure. The nasal cavity is divided by the nasal septum into two parts which have similar anatomical structure but may be asymmetrical.

The septum is a structure composed partly of cartilage and partly of bone. Anteriorly, the septum is formed by the quadrilateral cartilage. Posterior to this is the perpendicular plate of the ethmoid, while behind that the rostrum of the sphenoid bone helps to form the partition. Below, the quadrilateral cartilage articulates with the maxillary spine and with the vomer. The septum is covered with perichondrium where there is cartilage, with periosteum where there is bone, and superficially with mucous membrane (Fig. 9.2).

On the lateral wall there is a system of ridges known as the turbinates, each of which overhangs a groove known as a meatus. There are three turbinates: inferior, middle and superior. The inferior turbinate forms a bone by itself, attached to the lateral wall of the nose. The middle and the superior turbinates are part of the ethmoid bone. The turbinates are covered with mucous membrane that is, for the most part, columnar ciliated epithelium (Fig.9.3). Underlying the mucous membrane there is erectile tissue, which is found chiefly at the anterior and posterior ends of the inferior turbinate, in its lower borders, and at the anterior end of the middle turbinate. The meatii of the nose are of importance because they are the drainage channels of the sinuses. The appearance of pus in one of the meatii is of diagnostic importance in infections of the air sinuses opening into that particular meatus.

The posterior group of nasal accessory sinuses drain into the superior meatus and sphenoethmoidal recess. The anterior group drain into the middle meatus, while the nasolachrymal duct drains into the inferior meatus.

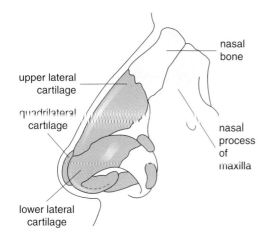

upper lateral cartilage

quadrilateral cartilage

lower lateral cartilage

nasal bone

nasal process of maxilla

Fig. 9.1 Anatomy of the nasal skeleton.

81

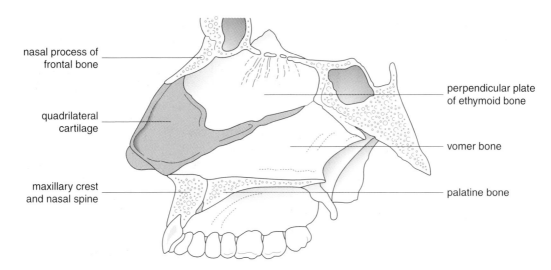

Fig. 9.2 Anatomy of the nasal septum.

Labels (Fig. 9.2): nasal process of frontal bone; quadrilateral cartilage; maxillary crest and nasal spine; perpendicular plate of ethymoid bone; vomer bone; palatine bone.

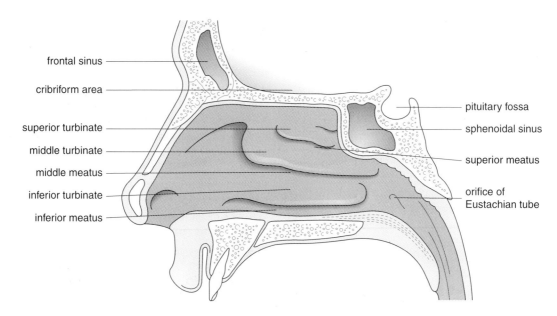

Fig. 9.3 Lateral wall of nose.

Labels (Fig. 9.3): frontal sinus; cribriform area; superior turbinate; middle turbinate; middle meatus; inferior turbinate; inferior meatus; pituitary fossa; sphenoidal sinus; superior meatus; orifice of Eustachian tube.

BOUNDARIES OF THE NASAL CAVITY

Inferiorly the floor of the nasal cavity is formed by the maxilla and the palatine bones. The roof of the nasal cavity is formed, in front, by the lateral nasal bones. Superiorly is the cribriform plate. This is a bony lamina of the ethmoid bone, which is perforated to permit the passage of the filaments of the olfactory nerves. Posteriorly the sphenoid bone forms part of the roof.

NERVE SUPPLY

The sensory nerve supply is mainly by the sphenopalatine nerve, the fibres of which pass through the sphenopalatine ganglion to join the maxillary nerve and eventually reach their cell station in the trigeminal ganglion. The sphenopalatine ganglion is not a sensory ganglion: it belongs to the parasympathetic system. However, a cocaine block of the sphenopalatine ganglion effectively anaesthetises the greater part of the nose. The anterior and upper part of the nasal cavity is supplied by the anterior ethmoidal nerves, which arise from the nasociliary branches of the ophthalmic division of the Vth nerve. These enter the nasal cavity at the anterior end of the cribriform plate and finally ramify on the outer surface of the nose as the external nasal nerves. Like the sphenopalatine, the anterior ethmoid nerves can readily be blocked by a suitably placed cocaine probe.

The sympathetic supply to the nose is also distributed through the sphenopalatine ganglion, which is reached by means of the deep petrosal nerve from the carotid plexus. The secretomotor supply of the nose is from the geniculate ganglion.

The olfactory nerves enter the nose through the cribriform plate in the roof and are distributed to the upper part of the nasal septum and the medial wall of the superior turbinate. There are about 18–20 nerves on each side.

ARTERIAL SUPPLY

The upper part of the nasal cavity is supplied by the anterior and posterior ethmoidal arteries, which are branches of the ophthalmic artery in the nearby orbit (Fig. 9.4). The ophthalmic artery arises from the internal carotid artery.

The lower part of the nose is supplied by branches derived from the maxillary artery, the most important being the sphenopalatine arteries and the termination of the greater palatine. Smaller contributions enter from the face.

These internal and external carotid sources anastomose freely in the nose. An aggregation of poorly supported vessels on the anterior part of the septum just behind the skin margin is known as Little's area and is frequently the source of nasal bleeding.

The lymphatic vessels drain posteriorly to the superior deep cervical group.

PHYSIOLOGY OF THE NOSE

The chief functions of the nose are:

- olfaction
- filtration
- humidification and warming of the air passing to the lungs.

There are other functions, such as vocal resonance, self-cleansing and the provision of moisture for the protection of the mucous membrane.

The functions depend upon the mucous membrane with its underlying tissues. In certain areas

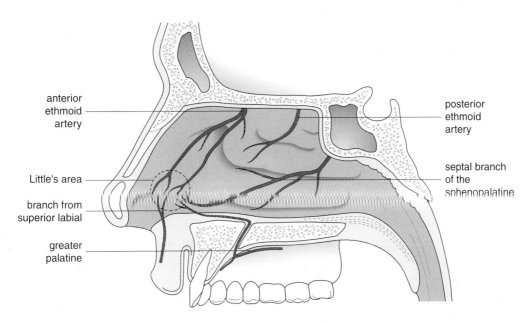

Fig. 9.4 Arterial anastomoses on the nasal septum. Bleeding commonly occurs from Little's area in young people.

such as the turbinates this is a complicated structure of ciliary mucous membrane, glands, blood spaces and connective tissues based upon bone, and is under the control of the autonomic nervous system. In this way the turbinates act as a valve mechanism, enlarging or narrowing the air channels and so determining the direction of the air stream. The path of the air column in the nose during inspiration is upwards and backwards towards the middle turbinate, thence in a curve towards the posterior nares. This can be demonstrated by the inhalation of a small quantity of coloured powder. In expiration such a definite path is not followed, but there is a more general diffusion of the air column throughout the nose, with an eddy round the middle turbinate (Fig. 9.5).

Olfaction as a function may be influenced in various ways. For example, obstruction from inflammation or vasomotor changes may prevent air reaching the olfactory area. Sometimes toxic or infective conditions, or head injury, damage the nerve endings and destroy or alter the sense of smell.

Filtration is effected by the adhesion to the mucous film of dust, bacteria and other particles. These are removed by ciliary action into the pharynx and swallowed with the secretions.

The moistening and warming of the air passing to the lungs is one of the chief functions of the nose. Air reaches the lungs at about 30°C and at 75–95% relative humidity. When, during cold weather, the air in a room is heated, the humidity is as low as 5–10%. To increase this humidity to the level necessary for comfort may place a severe strain on the nasal mechanism. Unless the mucous membrane is very efficient, extreme discomfort may result. Similarly, changes in the mucous membrane of the nose caused by disease or trauma may produce symptoms. These are the result of the inability of the glands and blood spaces to provide the warmth and moisture demanded by the atmospheric conditions.

Ciliary action is the means by which the mucous membrane cleanses itself and removes unwanted material. A constant streaming of mucus is produced anteroposteriorly by the movement of the cilia which fringe the surface cells. Any interference with normal ciliary action causes an

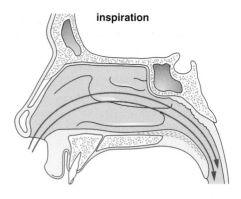

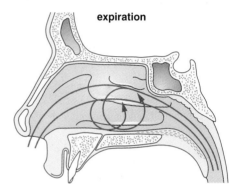

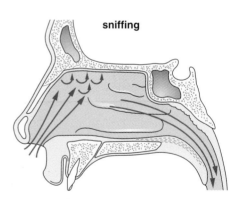

Fig. 9.5 Air currents in the nose during inspiration, expiration (note the eddy around the middle turbinate), and sniffing (note the eddies that occur high in the olfactory cleft to assist olfaction).

unpleasant accumulation of secretions or even the formation of crusts which cause 'drip', or 'catarrh'. This is often a source of complaint and is an expression of the inability of the ciliary mechanism to deal with thickened mucus, which slowly finds its way into the pharynx, where it accumulates. The conditions necessary for efficient ciliary action are mucus of the correct consistency and adequate aeration. Conditions deleterious to ciliary action are excessive drying, inflammation and thick secretions.

Treatment is therefore directed at restoration of the nasal airway, where impaired, and the production of conditions favourable to normal ciliary action. Any solutions used should be isotonic, and antiseptics are for the most part useless. Salves, oils and snuffs which slow up ciliary action should be avoided. Ephedrine used in saline up to the strength of 2% is a useful drug as it has no ill effects on ciliary action and produces little 'rebound' swelling.

The nose plays an important part in giving resonance to the voice. Malformations of the nasopharynx and obstructions in the nose itself may alter the tone of the voice, making it flat and uninteresting. In the same manner, by interfering with the nasal air column, rigidity or fibrosis of the soft palate may deprive the voice of timbre. For this reason nasal operations upon singers must be approached with great caution, and considerable experience is required in judging the probable effects on the voice of those treatments that alter the nasal structure.

PARANASAL SINUSES

The nasal accessory sinuses are air spaces which develop in the bones of the skull and communicate with the nasal cavity. The anterior group comprises the frontal air sinus, the maxillary air sinus and the anterior ethmoidal air cells. The posterior group comprises the posterior ethmoidal air cells and the sphenoidal sinus. This grouping of the sinuses is arranged more from the point of view of drainage than from actual anatomical distribution. The sinuses vary so widely in their positions during development that the distinction between 'anterior' and 'posterior' might be completely misleading. The anterior group of sinuses drains into the middle meatus and the posterior group drains into the superior meatus and the sphenoethmoidal recess.

Ventilation and drainage of the large maxillary and frontal sinuses occur through very narrow and complicated clefts before reaching the middle meatus. These two clefts in the lateral nasal wall are the

ethmoidal infundibulum and frontal recess, respectively and are parts of the anterior ethmoid system (Fig. 9.6). Most inflammatory disorders of the sinuses are secondary to disease within the anterior ethmoids, emphasising the importance of the anatomy of the ethmoidal bone and sinuses. The ethmoidal infundibulum is a cleft-like three-dimensional space in the lateral nasal wall. Its medial wall is the uncinate process, while the major part of its lateral wall is the lamina papyracea of the orbit. The frontal recess is a three-dimensional space bordered posteriorly by the bulla, laterally by the lamina papyracea and medially by the anterior portion of the middle turbinate.

Ethmoid bone and sinuses

The ethmoid bone is made up of five parts: the perpendicular plate, the horizontal cribriform plate, the crista galli and two lateral labyrinths of cells suspended by the horizontal plate. The ethmoid has only two surfaces, laterally forming the lamina papyracea of the orbit and medially contributing to the lateral nasal wall, providing the middle, superior and occasionally the supreme turbinate.

The ethmoidal air cells are divided into two anatomical groups, anterior and posterior, which drain respectively below and above the middle

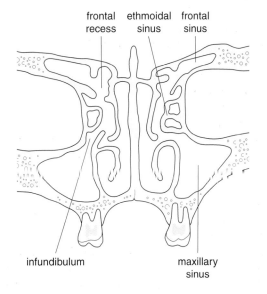

Fig. 9.6 Coronal section through the sinuses.

turbinate. In contrast to the other sinuses the eth-moids consist of very many small air cells without regular disposition, symmetry or fixed number. They lie in the upper part of the lateral wall of the nose. The middle meatus contains several structures of importance. The uncinate process is a thin, sickle-shaped bone turning from anterosuperior to pos-teroinferior. Its posterosuperior margin is sharp and concave and lies parallel to the anterior surface of the bulla ethmoidales. This free edge is not fused with any structure and between it and the bulla is a two-dimensional space called the hiatus semilunaris (Fig. 9.7). This space leads into the three-dimensional space of the infundibulum. The ethmoidal bulla is the most constant and the largest cell in the anterior ethmoid. The most anterior superior insertion of the middle turbinate is called the agger nasi, a region in which there is usually an aerated cell. The middle section of the attachment of the middle turbinate fixes it to the lamina papyracea; it runs in a frontal plane and is called the ground lamella, defining the border between the anterior and pos-terior ethmoidal sinuses.

All cells belonging to the posterior ethmoid open posteriorly and above the ground lamella into the superior meatus. All cells anterior to it open into the middle meatus.

Maxillary sinus

The fully developed maxillary air sinus (Figs. 9.8 and 9.9) should extend from the first premolar to the third molar tooth. The sinus reaches up to the floor of the orbit and thus occupies practically the whole body of the maxillary bone. Its medial boundary is the lateral nasal wall with the attachment of the inferior turbinate, while the upper posterior part of the medial wall frequently shows a bony dehiscence which is closed by membrane. This is known as the membranous part of the middle meatus and the ostium lies in this part of the wall. In addition to the normal ostium there is sometimes a small accessory ostium below and in front of it. It is important to remember that the infraorbital nerve traverses the roof of the maxillary air sinus and may be partly dehiscent.

In the floor of the sinus runs the superior alveolar nerve, and the roots of the teeth not infrequently project into the maxillary air sinus. They may be covered with only a thin plate of bone, in which

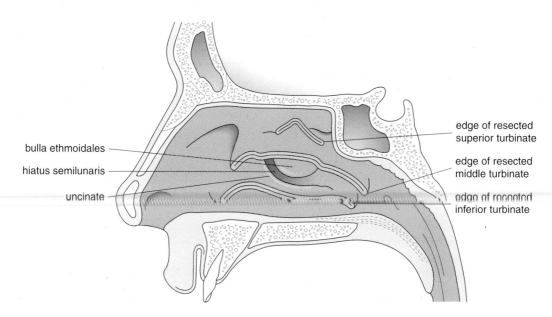

bulla ethmoidales

hiatus semilunaris

uncinate

edge of resected
superior turbinate

edge of resected
middle turbinate

edge of resected
inferior turbinate

Fig. 9.7 Lateral nasal wall.

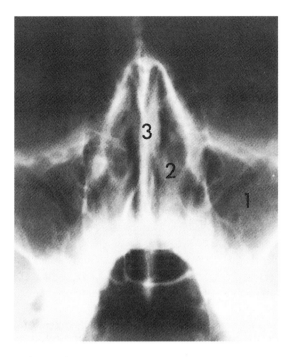

Fig. 9.8 Plain radiograph of normal maxillary sinuses. (1) left maxillary antrum; (2) nasal cavity; (3) nasal septum.

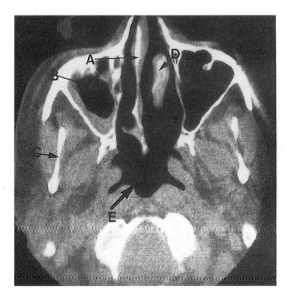

Fig. 9.9 Axial CT scan at level of maxillary sinuses. (A) septum; (B) maxillary antrum with some mucosal thickening on this side; (C) ascending ramus of mandible; (E) pharynx. The inferior turbinate (D) is included in the cut on the opposite side.

case the reason for infection of the maxillary air sinus in apical tooth abscess becomes obvious. Extraction of such a poorly covered tooth can result in an oroantral fistula. The anterior wall of the maxillary sinus extends as far forwards as the canine ridge; within the bone run small sensory nerves from the upper teeth to the infraorbital nerve. The hard palate forms a large part of the floor of the maxillary sinus.

The maxillary air sinus is lined by ciliated columnar epithelium. It is richly provided with glands, found chiefly around the ostium, which is situated high up on the medial wall. The cilia constantly beat towards this opening.

Frontal sinus

The frontal sinus occupies the space in the frontal bones between the inner and the outer tables. The sinus is not present at birth, but becomes the frontal sinus about the age of 5 when the air cells extend above the level of the supraorbital ridge. One or both sinuses may remain rudimentary, but when pneumatisation extends into the frontal bone proper it enlarges in every direction. The fully developed frontal sinus may extend to the outer orbital angle, upwards into the frontal bone for a distance of several centimetres, and posteriorly goes far back above the roof of the orbit.

The frontal sinuses are rarely symmetrical, and they are separated by a thin plate of bone (Fig. 9.10). The roof of the orbit forms the floor of the frontal sinus, containing, towards the inner angle, the supraorbital nerve and having attached to it, more medially, the trochlea of the superior oblique muscle.

Cells known as the orbitoethmodial cells are frequently found between the frontal sinus and the orbit; these cells may communicate with the frontal sinus.

Sphenoidal sinus

The two sphenoidal sinuses occupy the body of the sphenoid bone. They vary widely in shape and position (Fig. 9.11). They may be of unequal size and one may be almost on top of the other. The sinus ostium is high on the anterior wall and opens on

Anatomy and physiology of the nose and paranasal sinuses

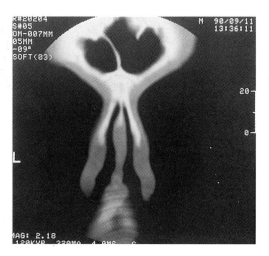

Fig. 9.10 Coronal CT scan of the frontal sinus demonstrating the asymmetry in size and the sinus septum.

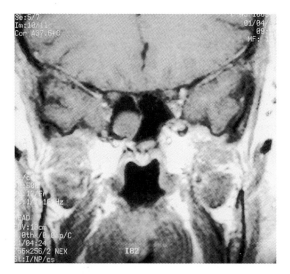

Fig. 9.11 Coronal MRI scan of the sphenoid sinuses. This scan demonstrates the unequal size of each sinus. There is a small polyp visible in the lower half of the right sphenoid sinus.

each side of the midline.

In most skulls, pneumatisation extends inferiorly below the pituitary fossa, which bulges into the sinus. Surgically the trans-sphenoidal route to the pituitary takes advantage of this, so that the sphenoidal sinus now provides the usual means of access for hypophysectomy. At the outer part of the roof the gasserian ganglion may form a superior relationship, while at the outer anterior angle, where the roof and the lateral wall meet, the optic foramen, containing the optic nerve, is in close apposition to the sphenoidal sinus. The lateral wall is in contact with the cavernous sinus, with the nerves and internal carotid artery which it contains. In the floor is the vidian nerve or the nerve of the pterygoid canal. As a rule this nerve is in the substance of the bone, but it may be lightly covered on the floor of the sinus and may even be carried in a bony arch across it.

> **Key points**

> ➤ The nasal axis is not parallel to the line of the external nose.
> ➤ The main sensory supply to the nose is the sphenopalatine nerve, which is a branch of the maxillary division of the trigeminal nerve.
> ➤ The arterial supply of the nose is from both the internal and external carotid systems.
> ➤ Little's area is an aggregation of poorly supported superficial vessels and is frequently the source of nasal bleeding.
> ➤ The main functions of the nose are olfaction, filtration, humidification and warming.

Examination and assessment of the nose and paranasal sinuses

A full history precedes clinical examination. It is important to identify the main complaint at the outset, whatever this may be: nasal discharge, obstruction, dryness of the nose or discomfort. This symptom serves as a guide for further questions. Ascertain the mode of onset, the duration, the character of the trouble – whether it is sufficiently severe to cause the patient acute discomfort or sleeplessness, for example, or whether it is merely an annoyance. The symptoms associated with the main complaint should be determined as well as a careful history of other organs such as the ears and larynx, for the nose is part of a complex mechanism, and laryngeal or bronchial complaints may accompany or follow nasal disease. The patient's previous history and family history are often significant; likewise his or her occupation and social history.

SYMPTOMS OF NASAL DISEASE

Nasal obstruction

This is one of the chief symptoms encountered in nasal and sinus disease. Nasal obstruction can be caused by:

- An anatomical or development abnormality in the nose, such as a deviated nasal septum or congenital atresia of the choanae.
- An abnormality of the mucous membrane causing hypertrophy, polyps or excessive and abnormal secretions.
- Abnormalities of the autonomic control of the mucosa, as in various allergic and vasomotor

disorders that cause episodes of swelling of the mucous membrane with sudden and often excessive outpouring of secretions.

Nasal discharge

This, too, is a common symptom of nasal and sinus disease: abnormal discharge may or may not occur with nasal obstruction. Discharge may be thin and watery, such as occurs with the onset of a common cold or with exposure to various dusts, pollens or irritant fumes. In more chronic irritation the discharge is often thicker than normal. Excessive accumulation may be the result of an overproduction of secretions, or excessively sticky secretions, combined with failure of the normal ciliary action which becomes unable to sweep the mucous blanket backwards towards the nasopharynx.

If infection is superimposed, the secretions may become mucopurulent or even purulent. Persistent discharge of yellow pus is usually indicative of sinus disease. A foul unilateral discharge in a child will often suggest a foreign body in the nose. Discharge of crusts in the adult may indicate an atrophic type of rhinitis. Thick, blood-stained discharge may suggest a tumour in the nose or sinuses.

Postnasal discharge, or postnasal drip, is a difficult symptom to evaluate. Clearly, however, the observation of mucopurulent or purulent discharge in the posterior choanae is important and may point to disease of the posterior group of sinuses. Very often, however, the nasopharynx appears normal in such patients, and investigations of nose and sinuses are likewise negative. Environmental factors probably play a part in the production of such symptoms – for example, excessive exposure to central heating with lowered humidity – but in many patients one has to assume that there is also a lowered threshold of discomfort, often with a superimposed non-organic element. Frequent postnasal hawking is a common aggravating habit.

Headache

Headache is not uncommon in sinus disease, and there are three basic groups of headache patients. Firstly, patients with headaches directly related to sinus disease, such as inflammatory disease, neoplasm or barotrauma. Secondly, those with pain that can be traced to non-sinus origins such as migraine, neuralgia or cervical spine disorders. Lastly, there are those patients in whom there is no obvious cause. The distribution of headache in sinusitis is highly variable: the pain can be experienced in the temples, temporoparietal region or in the occipital area.

Facial pain

This is a characteristic feature of acute sinusitis and barotrauma. The aetiology is largely hypoxia in the sinuses, although chronic rhinitis is also associated with facial pain. Stammberger postulates that afferent fibres from pain and other receptors in the nasal and sinus mucosa end up in the same 'pool' of sensory neurones in the sensory nucleus of the trigeminal nerve as fibres serving cutaneous receptors, and this explains the referred facial pain in chronic rhinosinusitis.

Smell disorders

A reduced sense of smell or its complete loss are not uncommon complaints in patients with nasal polyposis. The sense of smell often returns with medical or surgical therapy.

External deformities

Deformities of the external part of the nose may be developmental or they may be caused by trauma or disease. Maldevelopment may result in abnormali-ties of the shape of the bones of the nose. The nose may be deviated to one side or the other on account of unequal growth, or it may be narrow and underdeveloped, owing to insufficient use.

Injury to the nose leads to deformities such as the sinking of the bridge or deviation to one side or the other through displacement of the nasal bones. Falling of the bridge of the nose may be the result of a haematoma or abscess of the septum which has had its origin in injury. Cartilaginous destruction following injury removes the support from the nose, with the result that the bridge sinks. This same result may occur after a nasal operation in which more septal support has been taken away than the nose can afford, and a very considerable deformity may result.

Diseases such as syphilis, yaws and Wegener's granulomatosis are responsible for some of the most severe nasal deformities. The syphilitic nose is frequently known as the 'saddle-shaped' nose, with a marked sinking of the bridge and flaring of the nostrils, so that they look forward instead of down. Tuberculosis may affect the soft parts of the nose to such an extent that they may be completely eaten away. Cancer may also be responsible for extensive destruction of the nose and the surrounding parts.

EXAMINATION

The assessment of the nose and paranasal sinuses involves a thorough external and internal examination. Using a head light, the examiner begins by looking at the overall shape of the nose for the presence or absence of scars or abnormal swellings. The tip of the nose should then be elevated gently as this will facilitate the assessment of the vestibule and columellar regions.

Internal examination is best performed with the use of a 4 mm or 2.7 mm 30° rigid telescope (Fig. 10.1). The assessment should be performed in a thorough and systematic manner, and the first step is to get an overview of the nose. Septal deviations and spurs are easily noted, as are the appearance, colour and state of engorgement of the nasal mucous membranes. All areas should be examined: the nasopharynx and superior, middle and inferior meatus. A variety of topical agents may be used to anaesthetise the nose. Cocaine is one of the most

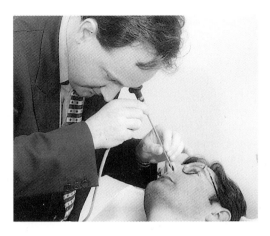

Fig. 10.1 Internal examination of the nose, particularly the lateral nasal wall, with a 4 mm 30° rigid telescope.

popular agents, as it has the property of retracting the mucous membrane to a very marked degree, and a 5 or 10% spray is often used in patients in whom oedema or inflammation renders a satisfactory view of the interior nose impossible. There are, however, many proprietary sprays which shrink the nasal mucosa very effectively without the possible dangers associated with the use of cocaine. One of these contains a combination of lignocaine 5%, phenylephrine 0.5% and benzalkonium chloride. The flexible types of telescope used today have largely replaced posterior rhinoscopy, which was probably the most difficult nasal procedure.

The healthy nose should present two approximately equal cavities or passages. These are divided by the septum, which is rarely exactly in the midline; the septum is vertical and broader at the base than in the upper part. The mucous membrane is smooth and pink and should glisten with a thin coating of mucus. In health, there is little difference in the appearance of the mucous membrane in the various parts of the nose. When the membrane has been subjected to abnormal conditions over a period of time, pathological changes are caused that enable the differentiation of those parts of the mucous membrane that have different functions.

The examiner should always have clearly in mind the order in which it is intended to examine the various parts of the nose. The exact order is immaterial, provided the examiner always follows the same routine. It is only in the practice of routine

such as this that the examiner can be certain that nothing has been missed; the following is suggested as a scheme whereby a complete examination can be rapidly carried out.

Examine the outer parts of the nose and vestibule. Place the patient supine and perform diagnostic endoscopy in a systematic fashion. It is important to avoid injury to the mucous membranes throughout the procedure. The first step entails an examination of the nasal vestibule, the nasopharynx and the inferior nasal meatus. This is followed by an examination of the sphenoethmoidal recess and the middle meatus is then assessed in great detail. Anatomical variants such as a concha bullosa, reversed middle turbinate or double uncinate are looked for. Accessory ostia, mucopus, oedema or polyps will all be clearly seen.

INVESTIGATIONS

Radiology

Plain sinus radiographs involve three standard views: occipitofrontal, occipitoparietal and lateral. They are today largely superseded by coronal CT of the nose and paranasal sinuses. Plain radiographs are useful for confirming acute maxillary or frontal sinusitis after demonstrating an air–fluid level. They do not, however, give much information about the state of the ethmoid sinus, which is the key player in the majority of chronic rhinosinusitis sufferers.

Computerised tomography (CT)

CT has become the primary radiological investigation for sinonasal pathology (Fig. 10.2). Bony and soft tissue detail are demonstrated and indicate not only the diagnosis but also the extent of the disease. The scans yield most information in the coronal plane and with wide bony window settings. Contrast agents are useful for delineating vascular tumours such as angiofibromas.

Magnetic resonance imaging (MRI)

This modality yields accurate differentiation between tumour tissue, inflammatory changes and retained secretions (Fig. 10.3). It does not, however,

Examination and assessment of the nose and paranasal sinuses

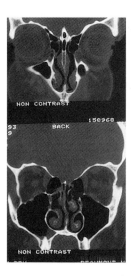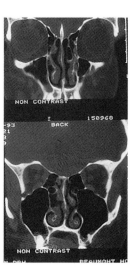

Fig. 10.2 Coronal CT scan. Four serial coronal cuts of the nose and paranasal sinuses using wide bony window settings.

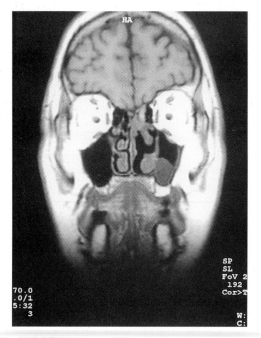

Fig. 10.3 MRI scan coronal view, showing a polyp in the floor of the left maxillary antrum.

yield a direct image of bony structures. Its superiority over CT lies in better soft tissue differentiation and it is particularly useful in tumour assessment. Both CT and MRI should be seen as complementary, not alternative, tests in the investigation of sinonasal disease.

Allergy testing

There are several useful tests available. Skin tests demonstrate immediate hypersensitivity mediated by IgE antibody. A number of common allergies can be tested – for example, the house dust mite (*Dermatophagoides pteronyssinus*), grass, pollen, dog and cat hairs and feathers. It can be performed using a scratch, prick or intradermal injection. Histamine is used as the positive control and any wheal greater than 5 mm may be regarded as 'immunologically specific'. This test is quick and easy to perform. The problems with skin tests are, firstly, that a person can have a positive result and be asymptomatic, and, secondly, that skin tests may remain positive for years after the cessation of symptoms. It is a useful test, however, and a large number of positive responses suggests atopy.

The RAST, or radioallergosorbent test, detects specific circulating IgE antibodies. It is expensive, time consuming and only tests a limited number of antigens; however, it is useful if the patient is so sensitive to allergens that provocation would be harmful.

Rhinomanometry

Rhinomanometry is an objective assessment of the nasal airway made by the simultaneous measurement of transnasal pressure and flow. Three different methods are currently in use for measuring the pressure difference across the nose: anterior, posterior and pernasal. In all three methods, the pressure in front of the nose is either the pressure inside a mask, if the patient is wearing one, or the atmospheric pressure in the room the patient is in. Active anterior mask rhinomanometry is the most commonly used because it has the least complicated equipment and is the easiest method to perform. Rhinomanometry can be used for the clinical evaluation of the symptom of nasal obstruction and for pretreatment and post-treatment comparisons for allergy challenge testing. Testing results in the simultaneous sequential assessment of the relationship of pressure and flow in the nasal airway during the course of respiration. The most important parameter reported is resistance, or the ratio of pressure to flow.

Acoustic rhinomanometry

Acoustic rhinomanometry is a recently introduced method for evaluating nasal geometry by an acoustic reflection technique. It is very useful for evaluating the geometry in the anterior and middle thirds of the nasal cavity. It is a method of measuring the cross-sectional area of the nasal cavity as a function of distance from the nostril. The principle of acoustic reflectometry is simple. An acoustic signal is produced by a source transducer in the distal end of a wave tube and this signal passes down the tube into the nose. As the sound passes through the nose, the waves are partially reflected and the transmitted signal and the reflection are recorded by a microphone and digitised by a computer system. Computer analysis of the signal yields a reconstruction of the impedance and area profile of the nasal cavity (Fig. 10.4). The area–distance function or volumes within the nasal cavity are then plotted. Rhinomanometry is the most appropriate test to estimate nasal patency, whereas acoustic rhinomanometry is more appropriate in assessing the geometry of the anterior nasal cavity and the response of the nasal mucosa. The two tests are complementary and should be used together in nasal assessment.

Olfactory tests

There is no ideal test for the sense of smell; there are, however, several useful and practical ones. Scratch and sniff tests utilise microencapsulated odorants presented in a booklet. The patient is asked to scratch a small patch and choose between four possible options. The advantage of this test is that it quantifies loss and can pick up malingerers. Normal values are available for a range of ages and both sexes. The disadvantages are, firstly, that it is expensive, and, secondly, that it has been validated from smells commonly encountered by an American population – not all of these odorants may be familiar to other populations. Commercial kits are now available of serial dilutions of a pure odorant such as *n*-butyl alcohol. This is a useful technique for assessing a smell threshold. Evoked response olfactometry similar to the auditory evoked response techniques still remains experimental.

Mucociliary testing

Mucociliary clearance can be simply tested by placing 0.5 mm of saccharin on the anterior end of the inferior turbinate – a sweet taste should appear in the mouth within 30 minutes if there is normal mucociliary clearance. If this test suggests a problem, the cilia should be examined in greater detail. Brushings of the lateral nasal wall, using a bronchoscopy cytology brush, are transferred to buffered saline. The ciliary beat frequency is then observed using a phase-contrast microscope and a photometric cell. The normal range is 12–15 Hz. The morphology of the cilia can also be examined using an electron microscope.

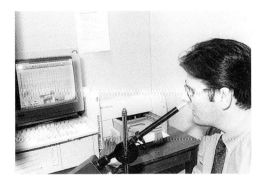

Fig. 10.4 Acoustic rhinomanometry. The acoustic signal passes down the tube into the nose and the reflections are analysed and displayed on a computer screen.

➤ **Key points**

➤ Nasal obstruction and nasal discharge are two cardinal symptoms of sinonasal disease.
➤ The ethmoid infundibulum and the frontal recess are two key areas in chronic rhinosinusitis.
➤ Rigid nasendoscopy is now an essential part of the assessment of the nose and paranasal sinuses.
➤ Coronal CT of the nose and paranasal sinuses is the radiological investigation of choice in chronic rhinosinusitis.

External nose

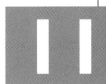

Skeletal injuries in the head and neck region are not unusual and may arise from accidental injury or from assault. Road traffic accidents account for most major injuries to the nose and facial skeleton.

Injuries of the upper third of the face tend to involve the frontal sinuses and may be associated with tears of the dura and CSF leakage. Fractures of the lower third of the face, that is, the mandible, usually require wiring or plating, and the more severe injuries to the mandible should be treated by a maxillofacial surgeon. Fractures of the middle third of the face require the attention of the oto-laryngologist. Such fractures may be confined to the nose, or they may involve the central segment of the middle third of the face – the maxilla – or they may involve the lateral part of the middle third of the face, which includes the malar bone and the zygomatic arch.

NASAL FRACTURES

Nasal fractures may be caused by accidental injury or assault. Fractures of the nasal skeleton can occur in isolation or in combination with fractures of the maxilla or zygomatic arch. It is important not to forget that the patient may also have received a head injury. The common nasal injury is a fracture of the nasal bones with or without displacement, an injury that may be compound or may only involve the bony structure.

If the patient is seen immediately after the accident, for example on the football field, and before swelling of the soft parts has obscured the deformity, reduction may be attempted; but if treatment is not immediately successful the attempt should be abandoned.

When the patient is seen after the injury, it should be noted if there has been any laceration of the soft tissues or if the injury has been of the frontal type causing the nose to flatten and spread laterally. If so, correction of the fracture should be delayed. Lacerations should be repaired; the surgeon should wait until the swelling has diminished and accurate assessment of the deformity is possible (Fig. 11.1). The optimum time to operate is about 10 days after the injury, by which time the bony fragments are becoming 'sticky'.

There are two treatment modalities for the broken nose. Firstly, the closed reduction method, which involves repositioning the dislocated parts of the nasal bones by manipulation. This can be achieved under either general or local anaesthesia. The second treatment option is open reduction, in which the septum is also explored and injuries corrected. There is still uncertainty as to the ideal treatment of a broken nose. The reason for this is the difficulty in

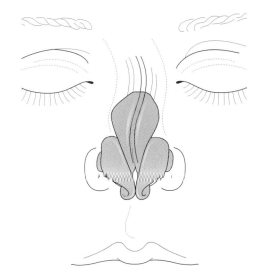

Fig. 11.1 Depressed fracture of right nasal bone with deformity.

evaluating the results following treatment. Follow-up should ideally last for at least 1–2 years because of late morphological changes in the nose due to scarring. There is also no standard way of evaluating results. Patient satisfaction does not necessarily correlate with objective morphology and function, and the pretraumatic condition has not usually been adequately documented.

Whatever type of treatment is chosen, a critical point remains and that is the unpredictability of the final result. In general, two groups of patient exist. In one group closed reduction will be successful and open reduction could be considered 'over' treatment. In the second, open reduction is appropriate and closed reduction may mean 'under' treatment. The distinction is based on the presence of septal fractures. A closed reduction is suitable for a unilateral fracture of the bony nasal pyramid with a stable nasal dorsum, or bilateral fractures without significant septal pathological changes. Open reduction, on the other hand, is more suitable for bilateral fractures with significant septal pathological deviation, bilateral fractures with major dislocations or infraction of the nasal dorsum, or fractures of the cartilaginous pyramid. It is important to realise that the mobilised fractured bony dorsum is in continuity with the upper lateral cartilages and the septum and is subject to the direct and later effects of trauma, such as buckling, bending and overlapping of fragments. Any corrective treatment must take into account the long-term position of the septum.

SEPTORHINOPLASTY

Correction of the deviated nose is far from straightforward. There are three basic perspectives in rhinoplasty technique: structural, functional and aesthetic. The techniques used to correct the crooked nose can be subdivided into four basic groups: surgery to correct the bony upper third; the middle third; the tip; and procedures to augment the saddle or depressed nose. It is the responsibility of the surgeon to balance the desires of the patient with what is realistically possible, given the anatomy and limitations inherent in each nose. Standardised preoperative photography is essential for surgical planning, long-term evaluation and medicolegal purposes. There are four useful views:

full frontal, lateral (right and left), oblique (right and left) and basal.

There are only three basic *incisions* to allow access to the structural components of the nose: the marginal at the margin of the lower lateral cartilages, the intracartilaginous (cartilage-splitting) and the intercartilaginous. There are only four basic surgical *approaches* to the nose: intercartilaginous, 'tip' delivery, cartilage splitting and the open external rhinoplasty approach. The goals of all rhinoplasty surgeons are adequate exposure of the tip and dorsum, access to the septum, as few incisions as possible, long-term security and avoidance of tissue trauma. The modern philosophy is one of preservation and reorientation of tissues rather than excisional sacrifice of large segments of cartilage and bone.

There is no such thing as a standard rhinoplasty. Each nose has to be assessed individually and the surgery tailor-made to the deformity. The surgeon thus has to be familiar with a number of different techniques, although there are several basic procedures that form the cornerstones of rhinoplasty. A useful approach is to perform septal and upper lateral cartilage surgery first, then to do the bony work and lastly correct the tip or augment. Septal surgery is described in more detail in Chapter 12. The septum can then be divided from the upper lateral cartilages, and this allows any inequality of the upper laterals to be corrected. The nasal septum can also be lowered in the supratip region. Correction of the upper third of the nose should be relatively straightforward. A dorsal hump often requires removal and the skill is in deciding how much to remove. Once a hump is removed, an open roof deformity exists; this is best corrected by performing medial and lateral osteotomies and infracturing the nasal bones. Medial osteotomy can be performed with a large 10 mm osteotome, while lateral osteotomy may be accomplished either via an endonasal or an external percutaneous approach, using a 2 mm osteotome (Fig. 11.2). The bones are manipulated to the midline and splinted in this position with a suitable external splint: the nasal tip may then be addressed. One of four approaches already described is used to access the tip. There are advantages and disadvantages to each, with no single technique being superior. Generally, the external

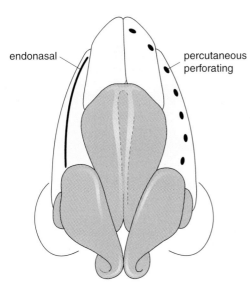

endonasal

percutaneous
perforating

Fig. 11.2 View of the nose depicting two different lateral osteotomy techniques: endonasal, and percutaneous perforating.

rhinoplasty approach is the best for severe deformities of the tip.

Augmentation is often required for supratip depressions or deformities. Septal or conchal cartilage has proved to be the best graft material.

Complications of rhinoplasty

These can be subdivided into early and late. The main early problems are bleeding, discomfort from the nasal pack, septal haematoma and septal abscess. Late complications include failure to correct the

deformity, supratip depression, saddle nose and bony irregularities on the dorsum. There are also several postrhinoplasty tip deformities. The 'polly-beak' deformity is a fullness of the supratip area and is usually a result either of insufficient lowering of the cartilaginous elements or of excessive postoperative fibrosis in the region just above the tip. They are complications more commonly seen by the inexperienced surgeon. Tip asymmetry, knuckling, tip ptosis and a retracted columella are just some of the other common tip problems after rhinoplasty.

> **Key points**

> ➤ Fractures of the nasal skeleton can occur in isolation or combined with fractures of the maxilla or zygomatic arch.
> ➤ The optimum time to reduce a fractured nose is about 10 days after the injury.
> ➤ Closed reduction under local or general anaesthesia is the treatment of choice.
> ➤ There is no standardised rhinoplasty. Each nose has to be assessed individually and the surgery tailor-made to the deformity.
> ➤ The steps in septorhinoplasty are: (1) correction of the upper third; (2) correction of the middle third; (3) surgery to the nasal tip; and (4) augmentation.

Nasal cavity and septum

RHINITIS

Rhinitis – inflammation of the nasal lining – may be caused by a variety of factors and these will be considered in turn, beginning with the infectious causes.

Infective rhinitis

Acute rhinitis or coryza ('common cold')

Acute infection of the mucous membrane with engorgement of the blood spaces results in a generalised hyperaemia of the mucous membrane, with enlargement of the gland elements and resulting hypersecretion.

Coryza is caused by a viral infection transmitted by means of airborne droplets. The disease is highly contagious and the onset of symptoms is precipitated by lack of immunity or lowering of resistance by chill, fatigue or similar cause. Increased activity of the normal pathogenic bacteria of the nose can then cause secondary infections which may lead to various complications.

The earliest signs of infection may be tickling, irritation, sneezing or dryness in the nose or in the nasopharynx. The prodromal stage is followed by an acute stage with copious nasal secretion. Some degree of obstruction may be present, the eyes are watery, temperature is elevated and the patient frequently feels a general malaise. Headache is often pronounced. After the early acute stage of profuse secretion the nose becomes more obstructed and the discharge grows thicker and more purulent. The general symptoms are improved, and after a period of hours or days the nasal passages reopen and normal breathing is re-established. The secretions gradually return to normal.

Treatment. As the disease is contagious, the patient should be isolated if possible and nursed in an even temperature of about 21°C with a humidity of 40–50%. If the patient can stay in bed, recovery is hastened and spread of infection to other people is less likely; sinus and chest involvement may also be avoided. Decongestant drops or sprays are useful in promoting drainage and preventing occlusion of the sinuses, as well as for the relief of discomfort. Ephedrine in saline can be used with safety, or alternatively a proprietary preparation may be employed, although the possibility of rebound congestion should always be remembered. Steam inhalations given a few minutes after the decongestant drops are also comforting, especially if combined with menthol or something similar. Analgesics may be used to relieve local discomfort or general malaise. Antihistamines are frequently prescribed to help decongest the nose and diminish watery secretions. Chemotherapy is not normally necessary but is of value in preventing bacterial complications such as sinusitis, otitis media and lower respiratory infections in patients who are predisposed to such conditions.

Nasal cavity and septum

Purulent rhinitis

Purulent rhinitis commonly complicates the exanthemas. Differential diagnosis depends on the specific symptoms and signs of the associated infection. The bacterial rhinitis which occurs is very often severe and more likely to develop complications than does the ordinary cold. Unless effectively treated, it is possible that purulent rhinitis may be followed by permanent damage of the mucous membrane which affects its functions later in life.

Treatment is the same as for the common cold, but should be more intensive and should always include antibiotics or chemotherapy with bacteriological control. Douching is probably best avoided. Associated sinus involvement must not be overlooked.

Membranous rhinitis

Apart from diphtheria, membrane formation occurs in pneumococcal, staphylococcal and streptococcal infection, especially in patients who are debilitated or malnourished. Bacteriological studies should never be omitted, and if the diphtheria bacillus is identified its virulence should be determined.

Treatment of rhinitis is the same as for the common cold. Nasal douching and removal of the membrane are of doubtful benefit. If the diphtheria bacillus is present, even if of low virulence, it is probably best to give antitoxins and isolate the patient. Chemotherapy should be used in all patients with membranous rhinitis.

Diphtheria

Diphtheria is now rare in most countries of the world except those in which immunisation programmes are incomplete. The nose can occasionally be affected, however, especially in children; it usually presents as a chronic serous or seropurulent discharge, which may be blood-stained and is often associated with excoriation of the upper lip. The patient is not usually severely ill and the condition may be overlooked. A greyish-white membrane covers the inferior turbinate and adjacent parts and bleeds when removed. A swab for bacteriological examination should always be taken whenever a membrane is seen in the nose and in every patient in whom any doubt exists.

Syphilis

Syphilis in the nose is now very rare. Primary nasal syphilis is exceedingly rare; it causes swelling and reddening on the affected side of the nose, rather like a boil or dermatitis. Secondary syphilis may be seen in infants in the condition known as 'snuffles', which develops in the first few weeks of life and is accompanied by crusting and fissuring of the nostrils. In adults it occurs as mucous patches with shallow ulceration and offensive discharge. Tertiary syphilis begins with gumma formation. There is swelling and tenderness of the nose with discharge, and the gumma later breaks down to produce an indurated ulcer with extensive destruction of the nose and foul crusting. The nasal septum will be perforated and the bridge of the nose collapses.

In congenital disease, lesions are those of secondary or tertiary syphilis, snuffles being the most common manifestation in infancy. Diagnosis is aided by clinical awareness and bacteriological methods, combined with a biopsy and serological tests in any patient presenting with a mass or an ulcer at certain sites, including the nose. Tuberculosis, tumours and various other ulcerations and chronic granulomas always have to be differentiated. It has also to be emphasised that syphilis may coexist with other diseases and can mimic them closely. Certain tropical diseases, such as yaws, can closely resemble syphilis, and now that international air travel is common and rapid, enquiries should be made about travel abroad in all doubtful cases. Treatment consists of local cleanliness combined with the management of the general disease.

Rhinosporidiosis

This condition is caused by a yeast-like organism, *Rhinosporidium seeberi*. It has a very wide geographical distribution, especially in tropical countries, but is endemic only in India and Sri Lanka.

Rhinosporidiosis appears as fleshy nasal polyps, often with grey specks upon them, which gives a 'ripe strawberry' appearance. The polyps are often pedunculated, and arise especially from the septum, but also from the floor of the nose and inferior turbinate. The complaint is of nasal obstruction combined with epistaxis and purulent discharge, which may be blood-stained. Histological examination is essential. Other nearby mucosal surfaces and skin are occasionally involved.

Treatment is surgical. Blood must be available because of the severe bleeding that is to be expected during operation, and endotracheal anaesthesia for protection of the airway is essential. Bleeding usually lessens when the pedicle is dealt with and the pedicle of origin is then cauterised.

Rhinoscleroma

This disease occurs sporadically throughout the world and is endemic in eastern Europe and South America. It begins rather like an atrophic rhinitis and then goes on to granulomatous formation. There is increasing nasal obstruction, with the formation of brownish tubercles which then coalesce to form a mass. The disease generally begins on the anterior part of the septum, but spreads to involve all parts of the nose, after which extension can occur towards the pharynx and the lower respiratory airway. After several years fibrosis and contraction occur.

The differential diagnoses are from syphilis, atrophic rhinitis, leprosy and other granulomatous ulcerative conditions of the nose. Diagnosis is made essentially on the histological appearance and identification of the *Klebsiella* organism in the smear.

In the early stages, treatment by chemotherapy combined with steroids for approximately 8 weeks can be successful. In the late stage with contraction, surgical treatment may become necessary, but the prognosis is poor and mortality remains substantial because of the laryngeal involvement. The antibiotic of choice depends upon the sensitivity report, but it is said that streptomycin is usually the most effective drug, oxytetracycline and chloramphenicol being next.

Tuberculosis

Tuberculosis of the nose is found chiefly in the anterior part of the nasal cavity – later it may spread around the cavity. It may involve the soft parts of the nose and the cartilages and cause severe ulceration and destruction. The bone is rarely attacked. The disease is nearly always secondary to pulmonary tuberculosis. The nasal lesion varies from a comparatively acute ulcerative form to a fibrotic type of slow progress, usually called *lupus*. Between the comparatively acute lesions and the fibrotic, many different degrees of activity are encountered.

The usual clinical variety of tuberculosis in the nose is the subacute form in which sessile granulations with crusting occur. They bleed readily and cause discharge and obstruction. Ulceration is frequently present and on the septum can progress to perforation. In lupus the disease is fibrotic in type and of slow progress. The 'apple-jelly' nodules that characterise the skin condition can be demonstrated if the nose is swabbed with cocaine and adrenaline solution. Diagnosis is chiefly by exclusion of syphilis and other granulomas. Clinical and radiographic examination of the chest is essential. Final diagnosis is by means of a biopsy of the nasal lesion.

The chemotherapeutic treatment of nasal tuberculosis is the same as that of tuberculosis elsewhere: it can be on an outpatient basis, provided of course that the patient does not have 'open' pulmonary tuberculosis.

Atrophic rhinitis

Atrophy of the nasal mucous membrane may result from a variety of causes and occurs in both young and old. Changes may be slight (rhinitis sicca) or severe, or there may be obstructing crusting with a fetid odour (ozaena).

Any condition that causes drying of the nasal mucous membrane will if prolonged give rise to atrophic rhinitis, which therefore may be occupational in origin. It sometimes follows nasal operations that result in undue patency of the passages; and a form, frequently symptomless, is encountered in the elderly. The aetiology is unknown. Early purulent rhinitis, chronic sinusitis, excessive surgery, endocrine dysfunction, malnutrition and, recently, an autoimmune process have all been considered as possible causes. There is a change from ciliated to cuboidal or stratified epithelium. Fibrous tissue is increased, and infiltration with round and plasma cells is marked. The glands are atrophied, the vessels narrowed and even obliterated; in advanced cases there may be change in the bone of the supporting turbinates akin to a rarefying osteitis. Similar changes may take place in the nasal sinuses, though these changes are frequently obscured by the infective changes produced in the sinus lining by the stagnant secretions.

The earliest complaint is a feeling of dryness in the nose, together with headache, commonly described as an aching behind the eyes. A feeling of rawness or dryness in the nasopharynx is not unusual. Nasal obstruction is often mentioned when in fact there is no obstruction present and the airways are wide. The feeling of obstruction in such patients is probably caused by the lack of normal airflow sensation in the presence of a dry, insensitive mucosa. True obstruction, however, may be present, because of the accumulation of crusts – these crusts result from the destruction of cilia owing to lack of moisture; the nasal secretions are no longer expelled from the nose but dry inside the cavity, with consequent crust formation and mild epistaxis when crusts separate. In patients with atrophic rhinitis it is wise to measure the erythrocyte sedimentation rate (ESR) to help differentiate the disease from that rare disorder, Wegener's granulomatosis.

The treatment of mild atrophic rhinitis is to treat the cause, if possible. Decongestant drops must be avoided. The use of a douche or spray is useful and can be made from a powder consisting of equal parts sodium bicarbonate and sodium chloride. A teaspoonful of powder can be dissolved in 0.25 litre of lukewarm water and used two or three times a day. Coexistent systemic disease, such as anaemia or malnutrition, may need attention; patients with severe atrophic rhinitis usually require regular nasal toilet. Crust formation is discouraged by the use of drops of 2.5% glucose in glycerine. In very traumatic cases temporary closure of one or both nostrils gives some relief, although no cure. Any concurrent systemic disease which is discovered, such as syphilis or tuberculosis, will of course demand treatment, and any associated sinus suppuration requires appropriate attention.

Inflammatory rhinitis

Wegener's granulomatosis

Wegener's granulomatosis is a multisystem disorder of unknown aetiology first described by Klinger in 1939. Three criteria characterise the diagnosis:

- necrotising granulomas with vasculitis of the upper and lower respiratory tracts
- systemic vasculitis
- focal necrotising glomerulitis.

It is now understood to be a spectrum of disease. The pathological basis is necrotising granulomas with a vasculitis, and infectious agents must be excluded. Although potentially fatal, it is not a neoplasm. The ESR is unusually high in these patients. Autoantibodies to extranuclear portions of neutrophils (ANCA, antineutrophilic cytoplasmic antibodies) are seen; there are two subclasses, C-ANCA (cytoplasmic) and P-ANCA (perinuclear). The patient with Wegener's granulomatosis is usually extremely ill, toxic and pyrexial, with symptoms and signs of upper and lower respiratory tract involvement. Urinalysis is usually abnormal and death occurs from renal involvement. The mortality for untreated Wegener's granulomatosis is 90% in 2 years.

Cyclophosphamide leads to a rapid initial response, and steroids with a daily low dose of cyclophosphamide are used as maintenance therapy. Steroids alone do not alter the outcome of the disease. Relapse is not uncommon and repeated prolonged courses of cyclophosphamide can lead to bladder cancer and sterility.

Sarcoidosis

This is a systemic disorder of unknown aetiology, characterised by non-caseating epithelioid granulomas. Nasal sarcoid is not as common as lower respiratory tract involvement, and when it occurs it is usually part of a multisystem disease. Yellowish lesions occur on the septum and lateral nasal wall and are associated with crusting. Septal perforation and saddling of the nose are not uncommon; lupus pernio can occur on the nasal skin. The differential diagnosis is between tuberculosis, leprosy, Wegener's granulomatosis and AIDS. Treatment is medical in the form of saline douches or steroid drops or sprays. Saddling is best treated with silastic implants, as autologous cartilage grafts tend to be destroyed by the inflammatory process.

Allergic and non-allergic rhinitis

Non-infective rhinitis is characterised by episodic sneezing, nasal blockage and non-purulent rhinorrhea. Rhinitis is classified as allergic when one or more causative allergies can be identified, and 'non-allergic' or intrinsic when causative agents cannot be found.

Allergic rhinitis

About 10% of the population suffers from allergies to extrinsic allergens such as animal dander, mites, house dust, moulds, yeast and pollen. The rhinitis is classified as seasonal if the allergen is to pollen or moulds and perennial if the allergen is present all year round, like the house dust mite. Allergic rhinitis shows a strong familial predisposition and individuals may present early in life with infantile eczema and progress to allergic rhinitis and asthma. In the nasal mucosa of the affected individual, contact of the allergen with cell-bound IgE produces a localised anaphylactic reaction, causing the symptoms of allergic rhinitis. The mechanism is as follows.

Mast cells in the nasal mucous membrane become coated with a particular type of antibody belonging to the IgE class. When the antigen, for example pollen, interacts with antibody on the mast cell surface, mast cell degranulation occurs. These degranulating cells secrete histamine and other mediators of anaphylaxis, including 5-hydroxy-tryptamine (serotonin), slow-reacting substance of allergy (SRS-A), platelet-activating factor (PAF), heparin and chemotactic factors for both neutrophils and eosinophils.

The immediate mast cell degranulation is responsible for the acute response, but a more prolonged 'late-phase' reaction, which develops within a few hours and lasts for up to 2 days, is common. This late response is believed to be associated with the eosinophils; T lymphocytes play an important role in promoting their migration, activation and survival through the release of cytokines.

The tissue in which the reaction occurs, that is, the target organ, may or may not be the portal of entry, although with a nasal allergy the two organs usually correspond. With hay fever, in which case the portal of entry of the inhaled allergen is the nose, the main symptoms are nasal. Less often, nasal symptoms may occur from ingestion of allergens through the alimentary canal; in food allergy the target organ and the portal of entry are clearly different.

Inhalants, seasonal or perennial, are the most common and important group of allergens in nasal atopy. Pollens from grasses, flowers and trees, as well as spores, characterise a seasonal allergy, so seasonal symptoms may suggest these types of allergen. Symptoms of a more perennial nature occur for example, with house dust. The house dust mite is found in high concentration in most bedrooms, as it feeds on skin scales. Epithelial debris from domestic cats and dogs may also be an important cause of perennial rhinitis, particularly if the animal responsible lives in the house or in close contact with the patient. The patient will often be aware that symptoms only occur in certain places and situations and this is clearly important in diagnosis.

Various types of food, but especially wheat and dairy products, produce allergic reactions. This type of allergy is much more difficult to identify and is generally the field of the specialist allergist. The nose can be the main target organ in some of these patients. Drugs, such as aspirin, iodine and antibiotics, may occasionally produce allergic nasal symptoms.

Symptoms In the acute form there is usually prodromal nasal itching. This is soon followed by violent sneezing and profuse watery nasal discharge. Itching and watering of the eyes are not an unusual accompaniment, especially if the allergen is an inhalant. Attacks may continue intermittently for days or last continuously for an hour or more, leaving the patient exhausted.

Chronic nasal allergy is not characterised by such dramatic symptoms. Persistent nasal stuffiness with a tendency to excessive mucoid discharge occurs, punctuated by lesser episodes of sneezing and watering. The differentiation from non-allergic rhinitis can be difficult. In children symptoms are not usually acute, but a clue may be provided by a history of previous infantile eczema, a tendency to wheezy bronchitis or a family history of allergy.

Appearances In an acute attack a pale oedematous mucosa with excessive thin, watery mucoid is typical.

Between attacks the nose may look normal, although in long-standing cases there may be hypertrophy or fringe formation of the mucosa over the turbinates, or polyp formation.

In chronic form the mucosa is swollen, but its colour is deeper red or even slightly blue, depending on the degree of venous congestion. The mucosa retracts strongly after cocaine application, and its secretions are not so profuse.

Diagnosis is in two stages: firstly, it is established that allergy is the cause of the nasal symptoms; secondly, the nature of the allergen is determined. At each stage a precise history is most important, and in respect of the former will include evidence of other allergic disorders in the patient and allergy in his or her family. A characteristic of the nasal secretion is the large number of eosinophils, especially just after an acute attack, when the mucosa is infiltrated with these cells. Other histological features are oedema and vasodilatation. To determine the allergen, history is again of prime importance. Skin testing with solutions containing various allergens is useful if skilfully done and interpreted in conjunction with the history. Of the skin tests available, the skin prick is more accurate than scratch or intradermal testing. Blood tests can show allergen-specific IgE in the serum (Ch. 10).

Treatment Avoidance of the allergen is clearly ideal. It may be possible in the case of feather pillows, woollen blankets, certain foods, plants, cats and dogs, as these may be removed from the house; however not every sufferer from hay pollinosis can take a long cruise during the grass season. Food exclusion diets may be tedious and demanding, but also dramatic in their results. The system generally begins with an extremely basic diet, into which various foods are gradually reintroduced.

Medical therapy A working group recently drew up guidelines for the management of rhinitis (International Consensus Report on the diagnosis and management of rhinitis. International Rhinitis Management working group. *Allergy* 1994: **49** (19 Suppl.) p.1–34.). The principles of good management are avoidance of the allergen wherever possible and anti-inflammatory therapy (primarily topical steroids) for prevention or control; this should be supplemented with specific mediator-blocking agents (primarily antihistamines) for relief – steroids inhibit or suppress many parts of the inflammatory process and topical steroid therapy is effective in prevention and treatment of non-infective rhinitis. Numerous studies have shown that nasal steroid therapy is effective in the control both of seasonal and perennial rhinitis.

In seasonal rhinitis, the onset of symptoms can usually be prevented if the steroid spray is used before the onset of the season: local side-effects resulting from the use of nasal steroids are relatively common but minor. Dryness and bleeding are occasionally reported, but long-term complications are very unusual. Antihistamines are often useful as an adjunct to local steroid therapy. All are broadly similar in the effective control of itching, sneezing and discharge. The first generation of H1-blockers (e.g. chlorpheniramine) had a marked sedative effect. The newer, second-generation antihistamines (such as terfenadine and astemizole) are non-sedating; however, there can be serious interactions with antifungals and erythromycin. There is now a topical antihistamine-azelastine hydrochloride-which may prove very useful.

Anticholinergic therapy with topical ipratropium bromide has no effect on the mucosa itself, but significantly reduces the output of the nasal mucosal glands. Potentially, it thus has an additional role in the management of patients with rhinitis in whom rhinorrhoea is a major feature. The cromones, disodium cromoglycate and nedocromil, have mast-cell stabilising effects. The major disadvantage is the frequency with which they must be administered: doses are needed 4–6 times per day to maintain their effect. They are also prophylactic agents and of little benefit when there is a well-established rhinitis.

Immunotherapy (specific hyposensitisation)

Studies have shown that immunotherapy is useful in treating rhinitis in patients with allergy to grass pollen, ragweed and dust mite faeces. There has been concern about its safety in the UK as there have been 26 immunotherapy-associated deaths over a 20-year period. It is currently recommended that immunotherapy should only be offered at centres where full resuscitation facilities are available, and patients should be observed for at least 2 hours after each injection. In the UK its main use has been in treating patients with life-threatening allergies to bee or wasp venom.

Non-allergic (intrinsic, vasomotor) rhinitis

In some individuals with rhinitis, no specific allergen can be identified. The symptoms are identical to those of allergic rhinitis; they are, however, provoked by non-specific exogenous factors such as cold air, humidity change, change of temperature, fatigue and stress. Cigarette smoke, air conditioning and central heating also appear to be common precipitating factors. It is believed that these patients have an overactive parasympathetic system. This hyperreactivity can be demonstrated by the individual's response to intranasal histamine, measured using rhinomanometry. Treatment depends on the presence or absence of copious watery discharge: when there is little discharge, avoidance of irritants (particularly cigarette smoke) and the use of topical nasal steroids are the main approaches. When there is copious watery discharge, the addition of topical nasal anticholinergics is usually recommended.

Surgery has a role if there is an associated septal deviation or turbinate hypertrophy contributing to the problem.

Drug-induced rhinitis

Alpha-adrenergic agonists cause vasoconstriction of both arteries and veins. They are useful for the short-term treatment of nasal congestion; however, a rebound congestion occurs several hours after use, requiring further use of the agent. There is also an increasing tolerance to the drug over time, requiring larger doses to achieve the same effect. It is not recommended, therefore, that these agents are used for longer than 7 days. Aspirin intolerance can lead to a rhinitis, and some affected individuals go on to develop nasal polyposis. Many antihypertensive drugs, such as methyldopa and guanethidine, can produce nasal stuffiness. Lastly, many drugs with anticholinesterase properties also produce nasal congestion.

Turbinate hypertrophy

The turbinates undergo cyclical increases and decreases in their size as part of the nasal cycle. Both allergic and non-allergic rhinitis can lead to pathological, persistent increase in turbinate size. This often causes a marked restriction in airflow through the valve region with a concomitant sensation of severe nasal blockage.

Treatment There are numerous surgical procedures described for the management of enlarged turbinates. Submucous diathermy has been the traditional treatment. The technique involves a submucosal coagulation along the length of the inferior turbinate. The symptomatic relief is frequently short-lived, however, often lasting for less than 6 months. Turbinectomy is the most reliable method of tissue reduction. The procedure is complicated by haemorrhage in 10% of cases and crusting is also a common problem. Laser turbinectomy has been shown to offer a more prolonged period of symptomatic relief, often up to 2 years.

FOREIGN BODIES

Nasal foreign bodies are not unusual in children – these consist, for the most part, of pebbles, peas, pieces of rubber and plastic and other small objects handled by the child. The site of impaction is usually the lower part of the nose. Symptoms are those of unilateral obstruction and discharge. In a child, unilateral purulent discharge is pathognomonic of a foreign body. Removal by means of fine nasal forceps or a hook is, as a rule, simple, although it may necessitate the use of general anaesthesia. The rigid telescope provides an excellent means of looking for a foreign body high up in the nose or posteriorly. In adults, foreign bodies usually take the form of rhinoliths, which are sometimes calcium deposits on pieces of gauze or other material which have been used to pack the nose in a case of haemorrhage. If these foreign bodies have been in the nose for a considerable time, a degree of atrophy of the mucous membrane will be observed when they are removed.

THE NASAL SEPTUM AND SEPTAL DEVIATION

The septum can be divided into anterior and posterior segments by a vertical line passing through the nasal process of the frontal bone above into the nasal process of the maxilla below. The anterior portion is necessary to support the cartilaginous pyramid, whereas the posterior portion has no supporting role. Deviations in the posterior septum can be removed without disturbing the support of the nose. The classic submucous resection operation is thus suitable for posterior septal deviations (Fig. 12.1). Submucous resection (SMR) can be done under local or general anaesthesia. The approach is through an incision in the mucosa on one side of the septum just inside the nose. The mucoperichondrium is separated from the septal cartilage, taking great care that no tears or perforations occur, and the cartilage is then incised in approximately the same line as the mucosal incision. Through the slit in the cartilage the mucoperichondrium is elevated from the opposite side of the nose. Nasal cartilage and bone are then removed and discarded in sufficient amount to ensure that the soft tissues fall naturally into the midline.

On the other hand, some form of a *repositioning* septoplasty operation is essential for all anterior septal deformities. Each operation should be tailored to the patient's specific deviation. The basic steps are, however, the same and include the incision, exposure, mobilisation, straightening and fixation of the septum. Nowadays, the surgeon can use a head light, illuminated speculum or rigid endoscope, particularly useful for posterior septal surgery.

A unilateral or hemitransfixion incision is used for a septoplasty. The septum is then exposed by raising mucoperichondrial flaps (Fig. 12.2). The next step is to separate the lower border of the septal cartilage from its osseous base, and reposition it in the midline. A strip of cartilage about 3–4 mm thick often has to be removed from its lower border (Fig. 12.3). The septal cartilage is then freed from the perpendicular plate of the ethmoid – at the end of the operation the septum should be lying freely in the midline.

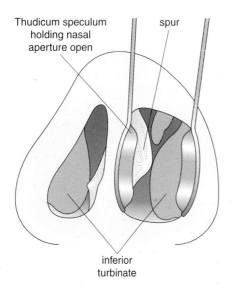

Fig. 12.1 Deviation of the nasal septum into the left nasal airway. There is a small spur on the opposite side.

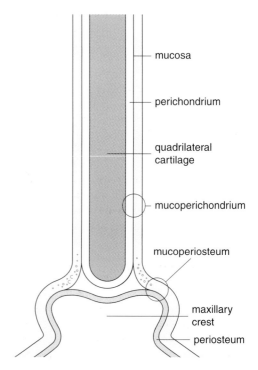

Fig. 12.2 Nasal septum in coronal section showing the relationship of the quadrilateral cartilage to the mucoperichondrium and the mucoperiosteum of the maxillary crest.

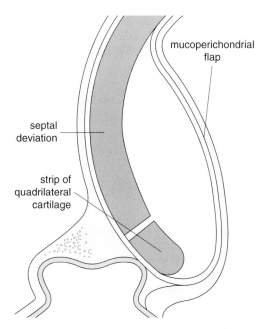

septal
deviation

strip of
quadrilateral
cartilage

mucoperichondrial
flap

Fig. 12.3 Septum in coronal section demonstrating the correction of a nasal septum deviation. The lower strip of quadrilateral cartilage is removed after raising a mucoperichondrial and mucoperiosteal flap.

Complications of septal surgery

Epistaxis is uncommon but may require repacking. Haematoma formation is rare but may necessitate drainage and repacking. Adhesions are more common in patients who have had combined septal and turbinate surgery; treatment requires their division and the insertion of silastic splints. Supratip collapse, saddling and septal perforation are more common after the traditional and more radical SMR operation.

Perforation of the septum

This is defined as a direct communication between the right and left nasal cavity via a hole in the septum. The most common causes are iatrogenic, primarily septal surgery. It is also recognised as an industrial hazard, notably among chrome workers. Chronic inflammatory conditions (for example, tuberculosis, syphilis, lupus erythematosus, Wegener's granulomatosis and atrophic rhinitis) predispose to perforations.

There is also an increased risk of septal perforations in patients with renal failure. Inhaled irritants are not uncommon causes and recently the illicit use of cocaine has been recognised as a potentially precipitating factor. In 7% of cases, the perforation is a result of malignant disease and biopsy of the edges is essential if the margin is irregular. Symptoms can be entirely absent but the patient may be aware of an irritating crust. Slight bleeding may occur when the crust separates; whistling sound on nasal inspiration is not uncommon in small perforations. Treatment depends on the size, site, aetiology and symptomatology. Asymptomatic perforations need no treatment.

Nasal douching is recommended when bleeding and crusting are a problem. Many symptomatic nasal septal perforations are satisfactorily treated by non-surgical closure using a silastic prosthesis; these are biflanged buttons. A large number of surgical procedures have been described for closure of septal perforations, and reflects the poor success rate of any one method. Surgical results are better for perforations less than 2.5 cm in diameter. A popular surgical approach combines an external rhinoplasty technique with a bilateral, bipedicled mucosal advancement flap, with or without an autogenous graft. The patient must be aware that the recurrence rate is high.

NASAL POLYPOSIS

Nasal polyps are greyish masses of pedunculated tissue resembling a bunch of peeled grapes. No single predisposing disorder has been implicated in the formation of polyps, although they may be associated with non-allergic (intrinsic) asthma and aspirin intolerance. Polyps arise from the nasal and sinus mucosa, particularly the middle turbinate, middle meatus and ethmoids: consisting of pale sacs of oedematous tissue, they have a poor blood supply and are usually bilateral. Nasal polyps are more common in men and their prevalence increases with age. Any child with nasal polyps should be regarded as having cystic fibrosis until proved otherwise. Any patient with unilateral polyposis should be regarded with suspicion; malignancy must be excluded by histological examination.

Symptoms

The major symptom is nasal obstruction, which is constantly present but of varying degree depending on the size of the polyp. Many patients complain of watery rhinorrhoea, postnasal drip and anosmia. Interestingly, facial pain and headache do not feature prominently despite obstruction of the sinus drainage.

Examination

In advanced cases the external nose may broaden. On examination of the interior, attention should be directed to the region of the middle turbinate. The polyps are insensitive to touch, mobile on their pedicles and may fill the nose bilaterally. Anterior rhinoscopy is suitable for advanced polyposis but rigid endoscopy is required to diagnose small, middle meatal polyps. Plain sinus radiographs are of limited value and, if any surgical intervention is planned, CT is preferable. If an endoscopic ethmoidectomy is to be performed it is essential. CT will demonstrate the patient's specific anatomy (in particular alterations by the disease process or as a result of previous surgery) and will show the extent of disease.

Treatment

As nasal polyposis is a disease with a wide spectrum of severity, treatment has to be individualised. Management often entails a combination of medical and surgical therapies. Surgery is not curative and patients must be made aware that polyps will often recur and that repeated procedures may be necessary.

Initial treatment will depend on the extent of polyposis at presentation. Small, middle meatal polyps can often be treated with topical intranasal steroid preparations. The most effective is betamethasone sodium phosphate drops in the 'head down' position. This can produce a dramatic reduction in the size of the polyps within 48 hours. Long-term maintenance may then be achieved with the regular use of an intranasal steroid spray. A patient with more extensive polyposis is usually best treated with systemic steroids. They are contraindicated in patients with osteoporosis, severe hypertension, diabetes mellitus, gastric ulceration or herpetic keratitis. Not all cases respond to steroids and some only achieve a partial response; surgery may then be required.

Surgery involves either an intranasal or an external approach, or a combination of the two. Intranasal surgery can be performed with a head light, a rigid telescope or a microscope. The intranasal procedure can range from a simple polypectomy to a complete sphenoethmoidectomy. Endoscopic intranasal polypectomy nowadays provides a means whereby most of the polyps can be removed with preservation of normal sinus anatomy. This is an important point, as many patients will require further surgery in the future. Endoscopic surgery requires a high degree of expertise to achieve good results with minimal complications. The external ethmoidectomy approach is now often reserved for recurrent polyposis where there are no sinus landmarks or there is distortion of the anatomy. Following either type of surgery, patients usually require some form of long-term intranasal steroid preparation to prevent recurrence or to lengthen their symptom-free interval.

Antrochoanal polyp

Antrochoanal polyps are a separate clinical entity. The aetiology is again unclear. The polyp has two components: a solid nasal one and a cystic maxillary one. They usually originate from the posterolateral wall of the maxillary sinus and extend by a slender stalk through the natural, or more frequently the accessory, ostium. Once through the ostium the solid polyp enlarges toward the posterior choana. It is more common in adolescents and young adults. Inspiration is relatively free but impaction of the polyp in the posterior choana on expiration produces almost total blockage. Antrochoanal polyps have a high incidence of recurrence unless all of their components, and especially the mucosal origin, have been removed.

Endoscopic removal is nowadays the primary treatment. The first step is to examine the maxillary sinus through the canine fossa. This often breaks open the cystic portions and allows removal of its contents, as well as any remaining cyst. The stalk and solid polyp may be extracted via the nose. It is sometimes necessary to perform an uncinectomy for an antrochoanal polyp.

> **Key points**
>
> ➤ Atrophic rhinitis is rare and treatment is difficult.
> ➤ Nasal sarcoidosis often leads to saddling and perforation.
> ➤ Wegener's granulomatosis is usually a systemic disorder and the mortality is related to its renal manifestations.
> ➤ Allergic rhinitis is common, with about 10% of the population suffering from it at any one time.
> ➤ Management of allergic rhinitis involves avoidance of the allergen, and medical therapy in the form of topical steroids and/or antihistamines.
> ➤ Septoplasty is the surgical procedure of choice for symptomatic septal deviations.
> ➤ The management of nasal polyposis involves a combination of surgery and medical steroid therapy.

Nasal cavity and septum

Rhinosinusitis

13

ACUTE SINUSITIS

This is defined as acute inflammation in the mucous membrane of the paranasal sinuses. Upper respiratory tract infections are very common and it is estimated that about 5% of these are complicated by an acute sinusitis. Many cases are probably initially viral, although secondary bacterial infection often follows.

The ostia of the paranasal sinuses are the key to the development of acute sinusitis – any factor which narrows the ostia will predispose the patient to acute sinusitis. Viral upper respiratory infection and allergic inflammation are the most frequent causes. There are two common clinical presentations: the first pattern is a cold which lasts longer than 10 days (viral infections rarely last longer than that). The second type of presentation is a cold that seems more severe than usual, with a high fever (at least 39°C) and a purulent nasal discharge. The patient with acute sinusitis usually has a mucopurulent discharge in the nose and the nasal mucosa is often erythematous. Facial tenderness is neither sensitive nor specific. Plain sinus radiographs are helpful in confirming the presence of acute sinusitis in patients with suggestive symptoms and signs, although the radiographic findings of opacification or mucosal thickening are not specific. The most important pathogens responsible for acute sinusitis are *Streptococcus pneumoniae*, *Haemophilus influenzae* and *Moraxella catarrhalis*.

Medical treatment in the form of antimicrobials is the cornerstone in managing acute sinusitis.

Amoxycillin is the preferred choice in most cases. There are, however, several situations where a broader spectrum antibiotic is appropriate. These include: (1) failure to improve while on amoxycillin; (2) living in an area with a high prevalence of beta-lactamase producing *H. influenzae;* and (3) the development of frontal or sphenoidal sinusitis. It should also be remembered that patients with acute sinusitis have a spontaneous clinical cure rate of 40–50%. Patients with sinusitis seldom require surgical intervention unless they present with orbital or central nervous system complications. Sinus washout may rarely be required to ventilate a sinus that has not responded to aggressive antimicrobial management.

Complications

By far the most common complication of acute sinusitis is chronic sinusitis, which is discussed later. This is especially regrettable because this complication is largely avoidable if the acute disease is properly treated. Complications beyond the sinuses may follow an acute infection or an exacerbation of a long-standing chronic sinusitis, and these complications may be multiple. As previously mentioned, CT is especially valuable in assessing such patients.

Orbital cellulitis and abscess

These conditions complicate both ethmoidal and frontal sinusitis. Three forms of infection occur,

Rhinosinusitis

namely cellulitis of the eyelids, subperiosteal abscess and cellulitis of the orbital contents.

Cellulitis of the eyelids is usually caused by ethmoiditis and generally occurs in a young patient. When the eyelids are separated it is found that eye movement, position, vision and conjunctiva are all normal. The treatment is that of the sinusitis and includes antibiotics: an abscess may occasionally form in the eyelid and need drainage.

A subperiosteal abscess develops if oedema and cellulitis progress to pus formation. Occasionally no sinus infection is diagnosed, or it may already be resolving. There is formation of pus under the orbital periosteum, generally in relation to the ethmoids. Movement of the eyeball may be impaired and the eye slightly proptosed and also displaced laterally (Fig. 13.1). Tension on the optic nerve can produce blindness if the condition is not properly treated. External drainage is a simple matter and consists of making an incision in the superomedial quadrant of the orbit and separating periosteum from bone until pus is reached. This is generally found without difficulty and a drain inserted. The cause of the sinusitis will demand appropriate treatment on its own merits. Endoscopic drainage is an alternative approach for those highly experienced in endoscopic sinus surgery.

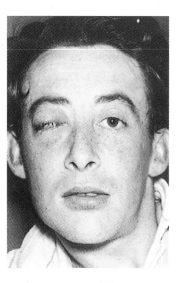

Fig. 13.1 Subperiosteal abscess. Pus has broken through the lamina papyracea from an acute ethmoiditis. Incision and drainage produced a rapid and complete recovery.

Orbital cellulitis is a virulent and dangerous infection which may prove rapidly fatal if cavernous sinus thrombosis and meningitis follow. Blindness is a common consequence. Infection spreads to the orbital fat and around the orbital muscles, vessels and optic nerve. There is severe pain around the eye and tenderness on slight pressure over the globe. When the swollen eyelids are opened, eye movements are found to be impaired. The eye is proptosed, the conjunctiva oedematous, and vision may be failing. The condition closely resembles cavernous sinus thrombosis but is distinguished by the presence of pain and tenderness and the absence of papilloedema. Treatment with antibiotics is of the utmost urgency.

An abscess may form within the orbit. Surgical drainage may help prevent blindness, which is otherwise a common consequence.

Meningitis

This is generally the result of direct extension of sinus infection but may occur from spreading thrombophlebitis. The principles of diagnosis and treatment are the same as those described for meningitis of otitic origin. The sinus responsible may be the ethmoid or frontal, and each demands urgent treatment.

Brain abscess

Sinogenic brain abscesses arise mainly from chronic frontal sinus infection. They may be extradural or within the frontal lobe and follow erosion of the posterior wall of the sinus. Diagnosis is difficult, but is greatly facilitated if CT can be carried out. This also enables the progress of an abscess to be monitored. Changes in memory, behaviour or personality are late and usually occur only in large lesions. Sinogenic frontal abscesses are mostly found in previously healthy young male patients. Referral to hospital with headache tends to be to a nonsurgical department, and the diagnosis is therefore delayed untill consciousness deteriorates. Treatment consists of repeated aspiration through an appropriately sited exploratory burr-hole. In the case of an extradural abscess diagnosed in the course of an operation on the sinus, drainage through the enlarged defect in the posterior wall is likely to suffice.

Osteomyelitis

This is a rare and dangerous extension of frontal sinus disease into the diploic bone between the inner and outer tables of the skull. Initial spread follows the venous channels as a septic thrombosis. It is not limited by suture lines. Intracranial complications are frequent and may be multiple.

Initial symptoms are minimal and the patient often seems remarkably well, even though there may already be a large extradural collection of pus (Fig. 13.2). A limited area of swelling and tenderness above the sinus ('Pott's puffy tumour') is soon followed by another similar area at a distance. Radiographic changes in the frontal bone are late; CT is essential to assess the presence and extent of intracranial pus formation. Intensive chemotherapy combined with drainage of the sinus may abort the early case, but if progress is not entirely satisfactory the scalp must be turned down and all diseased bone widely excised. This may expose a large area of dura, but this is not important and the residual

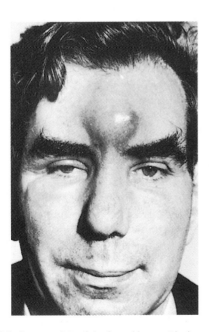

Fig. 13.2 Osteomyelitis of the frontal bone with abscess formation. It is important to recognise the significance of this type of swelling. The condition is dangerous, although the patient does not feel very ill. In this patient there was a large extradural collection of pus. Full recovery followed radical surgery.

deformity can be corrected later. Half-hearted measures carry a high mortality.

Cavernous sinus thrombosis

Cavernous sinus thrombosis occasionally follows ethmoid infection. The signs resemble orbital abscess, but the second side usually becomes involved, the retinal veins are engorged and the patient's condition is much more serious. The classical picture is now rare because chemotherapy modifies and masks the disease. Accordingly, the complication is often merely suspected; intensive chemotherapy and treatment of the cause now give a better prognosis to what was formerly a fatal disease.

Cutaneous fistula

This condition is only occasionally seen. Fistulae are usually situated near the inner canthus or eyebrow, although they may sometimes be on the forehead if they arise from a large frontal sinus. They may develop spontaneously, or occur when a subcutaneous abscess is incised – this may arise from the unrecognised empyema of the underlying sinus or osteomyelitis of the frontal bone. The treatment is that of the underlying disease.

CHRONIC RHINOSINUSITIS

Chronic sinusitis continues to increase in prevalence among patients of all ages, including children and the elderly. The definition of chronic rhinosinusitis is far from clear, although the primary complaint is certainly nasal congestion or obstruction. Other major symptoms are nasal discharge, headache, facial pain and olfactory disturbance; minor symptoms include fever and halitosis. Chronic rhinosinusitis has recently been defined as 8 weeks of persistent symptoms and signs or four episodes per year of recurrent acute sinusitis, each lasting at least 10 days, in association with persistent changes on CT 4 weeks after adequate medical therapy without intervening infection. Current opinion is that the distinction between acute, recurrent and chronic sinusitis should be based on the response to medical therapy, and only when it fails to respond to appropriate and aggressive medical therapy should it be classified as chronic rhinosinusitis.

Aetiology

There are three important factors which impair the normal physiology of the paranasal sinuses: obstruction of sinus ostia; impaired function of the cilia, and overproduction or change in the viscosity of secretions. Factors predisposing to ostial obstruction can be further subdivided into those that cause mucosal swelling and those that result from mechanical obstruction (Box 13.1). Certain anatomical variants in the latter group can narrow the already narrow drainage channels of the sinuses and predispose to chronic rhinosinusitis. A concha bullosa is an aerated middle turbinate; a reversed middle turbinate is convex instead of concave laterally; and a Haller cell is a cell along the roof of the maxillary antrum.

Diagnosis

There are three key elements in the diagnosis of chronic rhinosinusitis:

1. the history, as discussed earlier
2. the endoscopic assessment
3. the findings on a coronal CT scan.

■ Box 13.1

Causes of sinus ostial obstruction

Factors causing mucosal swelling
- Systemic
  - Viral upper respiratory tract infection
  - Allergic inflammation
  - Cystic fibrosis
  - Immune disorders
  - Immotile cilia
- Local
  - Rhinitis medicamentosa
  - Trauma
  - Swimming/diving

Factors causing mechanical obstruction
- Concha bullosa
- Reversed middle turbinate
- Haller cell
- Deviated nasal septum

Rigid endoscopic assessment has now become routine in the examination of the nose and paranasal sinuses. There are several important features to be looked for:

- the presence of pus in the middle meatus
- the presence of a reversed middle turbinate or concha bulla
- oedema and obstruction of the hiatus semilunaris, accessory ostia and/or swelling or bulging medially of the uncinate process.

CT should be requested in the coronal plane as this setting provides most information about the infundibulum, frontal recess and all other air cells. The scan should ideally be performed after adequate and aggressive medical therapy without an intervening acute infection.

The axial scan does not define the anatomy in a way useful to the surgeon and should be used primarily for defining disease in the sphenoid or frontal sinus. Plain radiographs are of limited value in the management of chronic rhinosinusitis as they both overestimate and underestimate the amount of disease located in the ethmoid sinuses, which are the key areas of interest.

ENDOSCOPIC APPROACH TO SINUS DISEASE

In the last decade many otolaryngologists have accepted endoscopic sinus surgery as the procedure of choice for the surgical treatment of chronic sinusitis. The technique as proposed by Messerklinger is minimally invasive endoscopic sinus surgery or functional endoscopic sinus surgery (FESS). The basic philosophy of FESS is to remove only the diseased areas in order to relieve obstruction and so restore natural sinus drainage, ventilation and physiology.

Surgical technique

The procedure can be performed under local anaesthesia with sedation, or general anaesthesia. Local anaesthesia is reported as being safer as orbital and intracranial complications are less likely. It is also reported that there is more bleeding under general anaesthesia. The type of operation performed will depend to a large degree on the extent of the disease as seen on CT. Before commencing surgery the surgeon should look at the scan and make sure that the lamina papyracea is intact and that there are no Onodie cells (posterior ethmoid cells often in intimate contact with the optic nerve). Anatomical variants should also be looked for together with the level of the cribriform plate and its relationship to the roof of the ethmoid, and lastly the extent of the disease.

The surgery is designed to address the *diseased* mucosa only. Normal mucosa is preserved. After adequate preparation and using a 0° 4 mm telescope, the uncinate process is removed either with a back-biting forceps, a sickle knife or with a powered instrument such as a microdebrider. The natural ostium is then inspected using a 30° telescope. Care is taken to find the ostium as 30% of revision cases are the result of failure to locate the natural ostium. It is important not to widen the ostium too far anteriorly as the lachrymal system will be damaged. The bulla ethmoidales and the agger nasi cells are important landmarks for access to the frontal recess. Disease in the posterior ethmoid is approached through the basal lamella. The sphenoid may then be entered either via the posterior ethmoid or its front wall. A detailed knowledge of the endoscopic anatomy and extensive experience of cadaveric dissection are essential before undertaking endoscopic sinus surgery. There are several important surgical principles:

1. Avoid bleeding and trauma to the mucosa.
2. Preserve normal mucosa.
3. Use cutting forceps or powered instrumentation.
4. Do not dissect too far superiorly or superomedially as the skull base may be fractured or entered.
5. If visibility is poor because of bleeding, abandon the case.

Complications

These may be classified as minor and major. Common minor postoperative problems are:

● adhesions

● orbital emphysema
● epiphora.

Adhesions are not uncommon, with an incidence of 5–20%, but only a small proportion of them are troublesome.

Major complications, although rare, do occur. These are:

● Blindness or partial loss of vision
● Double vision
● Meningitis
● CSF leak
● Direct brain injury
● Intracranial bleeding
● Death from damage to the internal carotid artery.

FUNGAL SINUSITIS

There has been an increase in the reported incidence of mycotic infections of the nose and paranasal sinuses. This is because of improved diagnostic methods but also an increase in factors that predispose to fungal infections; these include diabetes, immunosuppressive therapy and immunodeficiency disease such as AIDS. The principal fungal organisms causing chronic infections of the paranasal sinuses belong to the genera *Aspergillus* and *Zygomycetes.*

Aspergillus is an organism that is commonly associated with all forms of chronic fungal sinusitis in the immunocompetent patient. There are four different presentations of aspergillus sinus disease.

● *Allergic fungal sinusitis* is characterised by eosinophilia, nasal polyposis, mucin with hyphae on histology and IgG antibodies against fungal antigens.
● *Non-invasive fungal sinusitis* is defined as the presence of a mycelial mass confined to the lumen of the sinus cavity for months or years. This occurs typically in the maxillary antrum of an immunocompetent patient.
● *Chronic invasive fungal sinusitis* is characterised by tissue invasion, often resulting in bone destruction with extension into the orbit or brain. Invasion can occur in immunologically normal individuals, although this is rare outside the Sudan.

● *Fulminant aspergillus sinusitis* proceeds as a rapidly progressive, gangrenous necrosis of the soft tissue and bony structures of the midface. Patients at risk of developing fulminant aspergillus sinusitis are severely neutropenic. This illness often progresses rapidly and may not respond to aggressive medical and surgical interventions.

MRI is the best modality for identifying fungal disease. Ferromagnetic elements within fungal concretions give a decreased signal on T_1 and a very decreased signal on T_2-weighted images. The treatment of non-invasive fungal sinusitis is primarily surgical debridement and adequate drainage. The management of invasive fungal sinusitis in both the immunocompromised and immunocompetent host is similar: surgery and antifungal agents. Wide surgical excision of the bone and soft tissue is required in invasive and fulminant fungal sinusitis.

MUCOCELES

A mucocele is a mucus-containing cyst completely filling a sinus and capable of expansion. The frontoethmoid mucocele is the most common, although they can occur in any sinus (Fig. 13.3). The aetiological factors are polyps, trauma, tumours and previous surgery, particularly in the region of the frontal recess. Over 30 years can elapse between the

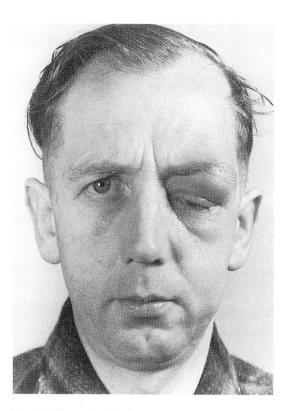

Fig. 13.4 Mucocele of the frontal sinus. Displacement of the eye was of some duration; the patient presented with symptoms of superimposed infection.

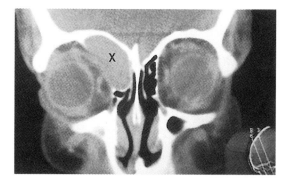

Fig. 13.3 Coronal CT scan. (X) frontoethmoid mucocele. In this cut the frontal sinus roof is intact, but much of its floor and the lamina papyracea of the ethmoids have been absorbed. The globe is displaced inferiorly and laterally.

traumatic event and the clinical presentation of a mucocele. Patients usually present with proptosis and lateral and inferior displacement of the eye and diplopia (Fig. 13.4).

Although plain radiographs may demonstrate opacification and bone erosion because of the mucocele, CT is important in determining the anatomy and extent of the lesion. It is now considered that most mucoceles can be approached endoscopically, although traditional surgery is still necessary for some. Patients without bony erosion and no previous surgery are the best candidates for the endoscopic technique. Lateral frontal sinus mucoceles may be difficult to reach endoscopically. The basic technique involves opening and marsupialisation of the mucocele with preservation of the mucocele lining.

> **Key points**
>
> ➤ About 5% of upper respiratory tract infections are complicated by sinusitis.
> ➤ Medical treatment in the form of antimicrobials is the cornerstone of the management of acute sinusitis.
> ➤ The three main sequelae of acute sinusitis are chronic sinusitis, and orbital and intracranial complications.
> ➤ Chronic rhinosinusitis is 8 weeks of persistent symptoms and signs or four episodes per year of recurrent acute sinusitis, each lasting 10 days, in association with persistent changes on CT, four weeks after adequate medical therapy without intervening infection.
> ➤ Endoscopic sinus surgery is the procedure of choice for the surgical treatment of chronic sinusitis.
> ➤ Fungal sinusitis is being seen more commonly because of improved diagnosis and an increase in predisposing factors such as immunosuppressive therapy and immunodeficiency diseases.

Epistaxis

14

Epistaxis (haemorrhage from the nose) affects all ages without sex predilection. Anterior epistaxis is more common in the child or young adult, while posterior nasal bleeding is more often seen in the older adult with hypertension or arteriosclerosis. The incidence is higher during the winter months when upper respiratory tract infections are more frequent.

CAUSES

The aetiology can be subdivided into local and systemic causes. Recurrent nosebleeds can also be classified according to the site of the bleed: anterior or posterior. About 90% of recurrent nosebleeds occur from the anterior septal region called Little's area, where there is a rich vascular anastomotic supply formed by end arteries. The two most common causes of recurrent epistaxis are idiopathy and trauma.

The common causes of epistaxis are shown in Box 14.1.

Local

Trauma

Any direct force causing a shearing effect or fracture of the nasal septum will more than likely be accompanied by haemorrhage. Digital trauma (nose picking) can readily damage the delicate nasal mucosa and initiate a nosebleed.

Inflammatory

Local inflammatory reactions as a result of acute respiratory tract infections, allergic disorders or sinusitis allow overgrowth of virulent bacteria and lead to dryness, crusting, exposure and haemorrhage.

Anatomical and structural deformities

Septal deviations lead to abnormalities in airflow, causing certain areas of the mucosa to be exposed

---

■ Box 14.1

Causes of epistaxis

- ■ Local causes
  - Idiopathic*
  - Trauma*
    - facial or nasal fractures
  - Inflammatory reactions (cold, influenza, rhinitis)
  - Anatomical or structural abnormalities
  - Intranasal tumours
    - benign
    - malignant
- ■ Systemic causes
  - Systemic disorders* (arteriosclerosis, hypertension, nephritis)
  - Toxic agents
  - Drugs (anticoagulants)
  - Blood disorders (leukaemia)
  - Hereditary telangiectasia

*Most common causes.

---

to constant turbulent air currents, and causing the vessels to rupture with the slightest traumatic insult such as rubbing.

Tumours

These are rare causes of epistaxis but should not be forgotten or overlooked.

Systemic

Cardiovascular

Arteriosclerosis associated with hypertension is a common problem, particularly in the elderly. The nasal mucosa is often atrophic and cracks easily. This eventually leads to exposure of an already arteriosclerotic vessel, which can easily rupture during a hypertensive episode, producing severe haemorrhage. Hypertension does not cause the epistaxis but ensures continued haemorrhage once it starts.

Drugs

Drugs can affect the clotting mechanism and must be considered in the differential diagnosis: some of the more common are warfarin, aspirin and non-steroidal anti-inflammatory agents.

Blood disorders

The clinician must consider the leukaemias, multiple myeloma, the haemophilias and idiopathic thrombocytopenic purpura in all cases of severe and persistent nosebleeds.

Toxic agents

Heavy metals such as chromium, mercury and phosphorus have been associated with epistaxis.

Hereditary haemorrhagic telangiectasia

This disease, also known as Osler–Weber–Rendu disease and characterised by abnormal capillaries, is a potent but uncommon cause of recurrent epistaxis (Fig. 14.1). The disease can also cause haematuria, melaena and cerebral haemorrhage.

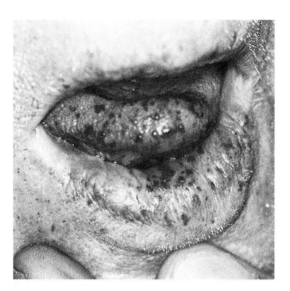

Fig. 14.1 Hereditary telangiectasia (Osler's disease). The epistaxis can be difficult to treat and severe; excision and skin grafting may help, as may laser surgery or embolisation. The lesions on the tongue and skin seldom bleed because of their thicker covering of epithelium.

MANAGEMENT

Arrest of haemorrhage

The nostrils should be pinched together and respiration continued through the mouth. The patient should sit upright to lower the blood pressure and lean forward slightly over a container so as not to swallow blood. Compressing the bony bridge of the nose is of no value.

Assessment of blood loss

A clinical assessment is made by recording the pulse and blood pressure. Signs of shock should be looked for: pallor, rising pulse and sweating. In cases of severe nosebleed, an intravenous line should be inserted, blood taken for cross-matching and administration of a suitable plasma expander initiated.

Determination of cause

A detailed history, either from the patient or relatives, will often illuminate the cause of the nosebleed. There may be precipitating factors such as trauma or surgery, or the patient may have haemophilia, hereditary haemorrhagic telangiectasia or von Willebrand's disease. Medical conditions such as liver or renal failure are associated with epistaxis because of an alteration in coagulation – the patient may be on anticoagulants and actually be over anticoagulated. A baseline haemoglobin, full blood count and clotting screen should be requested in all cases of severe nosebleed.

Determination of site

This is essential as the majority of nosebleeds are from the anterior septum and can be easily controlled with cauterisation or anterior packing. The patient is best placed sitting up, unless he has hypotension, and all clots are removed with nasal suction. A head light has been the traditional way of illumination; however, the 0° and 30° rigid nasal endoscopes offer a superior view of the whole nasal cavity. It is important to determine whether the bleeding arises from the superior or inferior parts of the nasal fossa or septum, as this information will be useful in planning definitive surgery should packing not control the haemorrhage.

Control of bleeding

Anterior epistaxis

Bleeding vessels or points on the anterior septum can usually be controlled with cauterisation after anaesthetising the nasal mucosa. A cotton-wool pledglet soaked in 5–10% cocaine with an equal-amount of 1:1000 adrenaline and squeezed out is a very useful technique. Very often the bleeding will have stopped as a result of direct pressure by pinching the nose or from the vasoconstrictive action of the cocaine and adrenaline. A search is then made in the clean dry nose for the responsible vessel. This is frequently identified without difficulty and can be cauterised with silver nitrate or electrocautery. If it cannot be controlled and the bleeding continues, a pack may be needed (Fig. 14.2). There are numerous different packs on the market, for example Vaseline gauze, bismuth Iodoform paraffin paste (BIPP) and commercially produced sponge 'tampons'. The specific one chosen is often dictated by personal preference, the surgeon's experience, cost and availability. Anterior nasal packs are usually left in situ for 24 hours, although there is no indication in the literature as to how long they should ideally be left in. They are uncomfortable for the patient and should only be left in as long as necessary to control the haemorrhage.

Posterior epistaxis

Continued haemorrhage despite an anterior pack is probably a result of bleeding from the posterior branches of the sphenopalatine artery and will necessitate the insertion of a postnasal pack. A simple postnasal pack is a Foley catheter which is inflated once correctly positioned. This can be performed without general anaesthesia (Fig. 14.3).

Continued bleeding despite anterior and posterior nasal packs requires a formal examination under general anaesthesia. Any septal deviations which might hide bleeding points or prevent adequate packing are dealt with. Obvious bleeding points can be controlled with diathermy. Nasal endoscopy may help to locate the offending vessel. If, despite a thorough search, no obvious bleeding site can be found, a more thorough packing of the anterior and posterior nasal fossae should then be performed. The majority of severe posterior nosebleeds are satisfactorily controlled with these measures and packs are usually left in situ for 24 hours.

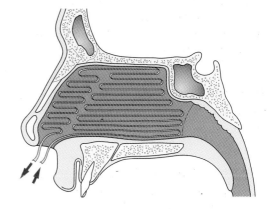

Fig. 14.2 Anterior packing for epistaxis using ribbon gauze. It is important that the packing should be built up in layers, starting on the floor of the nose and going as far back as possible, then gradually building up towards the roof.

Epistaxis

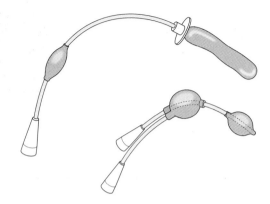

Fig. 14.3 Epistaxis balloons: ordinary and double balloons are illustrated. The latter occludes both the posterior and anterior nares. Air is injected using a syringe to obtain gentle pressure.

RECURRENT LIFE-THREATENING EPISTAXIS

If, despite anterior and posterior packing under general anaesthesia, the bleeding continues or recurs, some form of definitive control of the nasal blood supply is required. This is reported to be necessary in about 4–8% of cases of posterior epistaxis. In some cases, where expertise is available, this can be achieved by embolisation of the bleeding vessel under radiological control. Three main surgical procedures are described to control severe epistaxis:

● anterior ethmoidal artery ligation
● maxillary artery ligation
● external carotid artery ligation.

Anterior ethmoidal artery ligation

This is the least effective method as the artery only supplies 10% of the nasal cavity. It is most useful for bleeding that occurs in the superior part of the nasal fossae, the region the artery supplies.

Internal maxillary artery ligation

Ligation of this artery results in a decrease in the pressure gradient within the bleeding vessel, allowing a clot to form by the normal intrinsic clotting mechanisms. It is performed via a Caldwell–Luc approach.

External carotid artery ligation

This is quicker and technically easier than internal maxillary artery ligation. The decision to perform a maxillary artery ligation or an external carotid artery ligation will depend on the experience and preference of the otolaryngologist.

> **Key points**

➤ Epistaxis affects all ages.
➤ Epistaxis can be life-threatening.
➤ The two common causes are idiopathy and trauma.
➤ Systemic disorders are rare but should not be overlooked.
➤ The majority of nosebleeds are from the anterior septum and can easily be controlled with cauterisation or anterior nasal packing.
➤ Surgical ligation of the arterial supply of the nose may be necessary in severe cases.

Tumours of the nose and paranasal sinuses

Tumours of the nose and paranasal sinuses can be subdivided into benign, intermediate and malignant, depending on their behaviour. Tumours of the skin of the nose are probably the most common of the facial cancers; malignancy of the nose and paranasal sinuses is however uncommon, with an incidence of about 10 per million of the population in the USA and the UK.

BENIGN TUMOURS

Squamous papillomas are not uncommon in the vestibule, and simple excision is all that is required. Osteomas are benign bony tumours containing mature bone. They occur, in order of frequency, in the frontal, ethmoid and maxillary sinuses (Fig. 15.1). Their surgical management depends on their site. Frontal sinus osteomas are often pedicled and easily removed. Ethmoid osteomas, on the other hand, are difficult to remove and the large ones are better excised using a craniofacial approach.

Haemangiomas are not uncommon on the nasal septum. They are nearly always benign and usually no treatment is necessary.

Angiofibroma is a rare condition. It is a tumour of angiomatous tissue and fibrous stroma. The tumour is histologically benign but expands locally and may involve the ethmoids, the sphenoid, the orbit and skull base. The classic presentation is an adolescent male with nasal obstruction and bleeding. Computerised tomography with contrast has eliminated the need for, and the risk of, biopsy. Surgery is the treatment of choice but should be avoided in favour of radiotherapy in cases with cavernous sinus encroachment and when there are parasellar feeding vessels from the internal carotid artery.

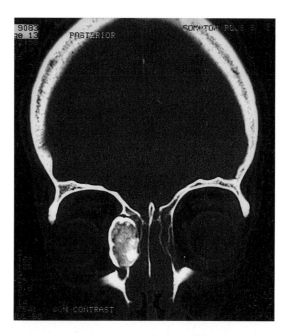

Fig. 15.1 Coronal CT scan showing a large osteoma in the right ethmoid sinus.

FIBROUS DYSPLASIA

Fibrous dysplasia is a skeletal disorder wherein medullary bone is replaced by fibro-osseous tissue. Monostotic fibrous dysplasia is the term applied when the disease is confined to one bone; it accounts for 70–80% of all cases. Most cases occur before the age of 20 and swelling of the maxilla is the most common feature. Excision or curettage is indicated only if the lesion interferes with function, progresses indefinitely or undergoes sarcomatous change. The primary goal is contouring to minimise deformity.

INTERMEDIATE TUMOURS

Inverting papilloma

This lesion represents about 4% of all nasal neoplasms. Males are affected three times more frequently than females. The tumour commonly arises in the lateral wall of the nose and presents as a unilateral nasal polyp.

The lesion is characterised by being locally aggressive and causing bony erosion of the lateral nasal wall (Fig. 15.2). An inverting papilloma has a high propensity for recurrence after removal and is also associated with a synchronous malignancy in 15% of cases. This fact highlights the importance of sending polyp tissue for histology, particularly if it is unilateral. Treatment is aimed at removal of the tumour, without mutilation, and at detecting malignancy. A lateral rhinotomy is the approach most often used.

MALIGNANT TUMOURS

These tumours, unlike most of the other head and neck cancers, do not usually occur in the heavy smoking or heavy drinking population. They may occasionally result from exposure to environmental carcinogens. For example, woodworkers are at increased risk of developing adenocarcinoma of the sinuses. The maxillary sinus is the most common site for development of malignancy (Fig. 15.3). Squamous carcinoma is the most common malignancy and is twice as common in men as in women. Other less frequent tumours are adenocarcinoma, malignant melanoma, ethesioneuroblastoma, sarcoma and lymphoma. The average age at presentation is 60 and squamous carcinoma rarely occurs under the age of 40.

The chief symptoms of a nasal tumour are unilateral obstruction with haemorrhage or a purulent and sanguineous discharge. Broadening of the nasal bones may also occur as the tumour increases in bulk. Headache is a late complaint.

The treatment of these tumours depends on their site, size and histology as well as the CT and MRI findings. There are at least four commonly employed staging systems. All regard bony invasion of the maxillary suprastructure posteriorly and/or superiorly as indicating a poorer prognosis than tumours which invade bone anteriorly and inferiorly. The site and size of the tumour will dictate the surgical approach. The standard approach is a radical maxillectomy, as the maxillary sinus is the most

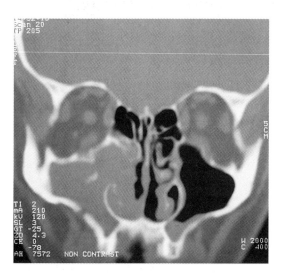

Fig. 15.2 Coronal CT scan. An inverting papilloma fills the antrum on the right and the adjacent nose. There is bony erosion of the lateral nasal wall. Compare the normal structures on the opposite side.

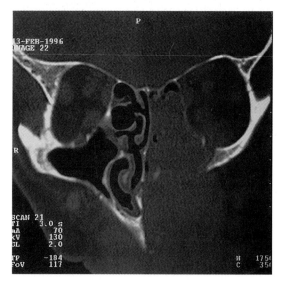

Fig. 15.3 Coronal CT scan. The maxillary antrum on the left is filled with tumour which has destroyed its inferior wall and invaded the hard palate and soft tissues of the cheek.

common site. Tumours involving the superior ethmoid complex and/or the cribriform plate are best removed via a craniofacial excision. Collaboration with other specialists is essential in formulating a treatment strategy. An ophthalmological opinion is important in determining any extension into the ipsilateral eye – it is also necessary to know the status of the contralateral eye. The oral surgeon and prosthodontist are important members of the team, especially in the reconstruction of the oral cavity defect (Fig. 15.4).

Before embarking on a major surgical procedure, it is essential to establish whether or not the tumour can be safely removed. The main contraindications to surgery are posterior extensions into the sphenoid sinus, involvement of both optic nerves, invasion of the middle cranial fossa, extension into the nasopharynx and distant metastatic disease. Postoperative radiotherapy is recommended for most malignant tumours of the ethmoid region and for the majority of tumours of the maxillary sinus where there are microscopically positive margins or perineural invasion is present. Chemotherapy offers no benefit in cases of squamous carcinoma, either as part of definitive treatment or in palliation. Only too frequently it merely adds to the patient's misery.

T CELL LYMPHOMA ('MIDLINE', 'MALIGNANT', 'LETHAL' GRANULOMA)

The term 'malignant' or 'lethal' midline granuloma is no longer justified for this slowly progressive, ulcerative, destructive lesion of the tissues of the nose, sinuses and face, although severe mutilation occurs, and death follows if the condition is not

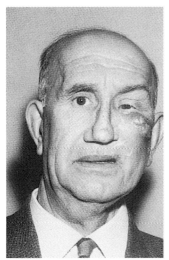

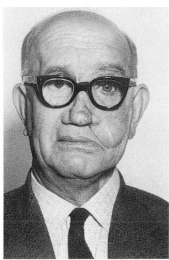

Fig. 15.4 A suitable prosthesis can be made to cover a surgical defect. This one followed surgical treatment of a carcinoma of the antrum.

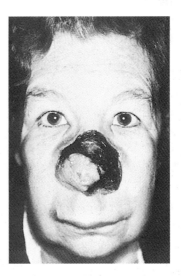

Fig. 15.5 This lesion began as something resembling a small pimple. The nose gradually mummified and fell off a few days after this photograph was taken. The diagnosis is midline granuloma. The patient was well 9 years after excision of necrotic tissue followed by radiotherapy. A prosthesis covered the defect very satisfactorily.

Tumours of the nose and paranasal sinuses

controlled. There has been much discussion about the aetiology of this curious disease, which is now regarded as a T cell lymphoma. The rate of destruction varies substantially from patient to patient, probably being influenced by the patient's own immunological reactions. Systemic disease occasionally occurs in the form of malignant lymphomas (Fig. 15.5). Histological diagnosis is seldom straightforward, mainly because of the amount of necrosis and infection present in any biopsy material. A report of non-specific inflammatory granulation tissue is an indication that further biopsies should be made, and such a report in tissue obtained from a progressive destructive lesion in the region of the nose or sinuses should raise the suspicion of midline granuloma. The condition responds well to radiotherapy in full doses. Antibiotics may be used for coexistent infection. Surgical excision should be limited to simple removal of necrotic tissue.

> **Key points**

- ➤ Malignancy of the nose and paranasal sinuses is rare.
- ➤ Squamous papilloma is a common benign tumour.
- ➤ Inverting papilloma has a high propensity for recurrence and is associated with a synchronous malignancy in about 15% of cases.
- ➤ All unilateral polyps should be submitted for histology to rule out malignancy.
- ➤ The maxillary sinus is the most common site of malignancy.
- ➤ Squamous carcinoma is the most common malignant tumour.
- ➤ Treatment depends on the site, size and histology but usually involves a combination of surgery and postoperative radiotherapy.

THE NECK 3

Anatomy and examination of the neck

The neck is an anatomically complex area. A sound knowledge of this anatomy is essential to an understanding of the various disorders of the structures that it constitutes. Certain neck swellings may be diagnosed purely on anatomical grounds because of their site, for example a thyroid or parotid swelling. Patients may complain of swellings which are abnormal; they sometimes become anxious about 'lumps', which are in fact normal parts of the anatomy that they have discovered by chance or that may be more prominent than average on one or other side.

GENERAL TOPOGRAPHY; ANTERIOR AND POSTERIOR TRIANGLES

The neck comprises an anterior and posterior part. Posterior to the prevertebral fascia lie the cervical spine and prevertebral muscles, which form the floor of the posterior triangle. The muscles attaching to the posterior part of the spine are bulky but of little clinical importance. Condensations of fascia form distinct anatomical compartments in the neck which are relevant in the spread of infection through the neck (Fig. 16.1).

The pharynx, larynx and trachea form a midline group of organs whose anatomy is discussed in the relevant chapters. The thyroid gland is a bilobed structure attached to the upper part of the trachea by the fibrous ligament of Berry and covered by the strap muscles. It is invested by pretracheal fascia, and its attachment to the trachea explains why it moves up and down on swallowing. Each lobe is intimately related posteriorly to the recurrent laryngeal nerves and parathyroid glands.

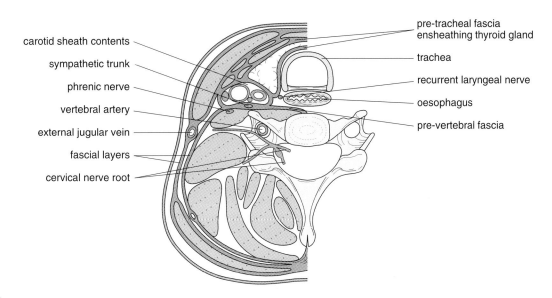

carotid sheath contents
sympathetic trunk
phrenic nerve
vertebral artery
external jugular vein
fascial layers
cervical nerve root

pre-tracheal fascia ensheathing thyroid gland
trachea
recurrent laryngeal nerve
oesophagus
pre-vertebral fascia

Fig. 16.1 Cross-section of the neck.

The lateral compartments of the neck are divided descriptively into the anterior and posterior triangles, separated by the sternocleidomastoid muscle. The anterior triangle contains the submandibular gland, thyroid gland, lymph nodes and the upper part of the carotid sheath. The posterior triangle is bounded posteriorly by the anterior border of trapezius. Apart from lymph nodes, the most important structure in the posterior triangle is the spinal accessory nerve, which passes through the triangle. Its clinical importance lies in the fact that it is easily damaged if a lymph node is biopsied in this region, leading to considerable morbidity in the form of a frozen shoulder. Its surface marking can be demonstrated by palpating the lateral mass of the atlas (where the nerve lies on the jugular vein) and marking a vertical line to the shoulder, with the subject viewed in accurate lateral profile.

The nerve supply of the skin of the neck is derived from the cervical plexus (C2–4). The sensory branches from the plexus pass behind the sterno-cleidomastoid muscle. The phrenic nerve is another, deeper branch of the plexus. It is at risk in neck dissections, until the point at which sensory branches are divided, because it may be 'tented up' by traction on the sternocleidomastoid muscle. The blood supply of the skin is derived posteriorly in a segmental fashion. This is important in the design of incisions for radical neck dissection – especially if previous radiotherapy has been employed – because an injudicious incision may lead to ischaemic necrosis of the skin.

The carotid sheath lies for the most part under cover of the sternocleidomastoid muscle. Its contents are the carotid arteries, the internal jugular vein, the vagus nerve and lymphatics. The sympathetic trunk and its ganglia lie behind the carotid sheath. The common carotid artery divides into the internal and external carotid arteries at the level of C4. The former is devoid of branches – a useful point in distinguishing it from the external carotid artery.

LYMPHATIC ANATOMY

A knowledge of lymphatic drainage is important. In squamous cell carcinoma of the head and neck the presence and level of nodal metastases is of profound prognostic significance. The lymphatic drainage from different sites in the upper aerodigestive tract is highly predictable; for example, the tonsil drains to jugulodigastric nodes. Most lymphatics are situated in the carotid sheath and therefore lie underneath the sternocleidomastoid muscle. However, important lymph node groups lie in the submandibular region, the posterior triangle (to where nasopharyngeal carcinoma commonly metastasises) and the retropharyngeal space. Because of the prognostic significance of lymphatic metastases, a classification of lymphatic groups into six levels of nodal involvement has been widely adopted as an aid to disease staging (Fig. 16.2).

EXAMINATION

Examination of the neck should be performed in a systematic manner, beginning with inspection from the front. Palpation is best carried out from behind the patient. Normal structures, such as the mandible, hyoid bone, larynx, mastoid process and clavicle, are readily identified. Palpation commences with the posterior triangle. The structures of the carotid sheath, including the lymphatics, can be palpated more easily if the sternocleidomastoid muscle is relaxed. The submandibular glands are usually palpable when normal, but the thyroid gland is not.

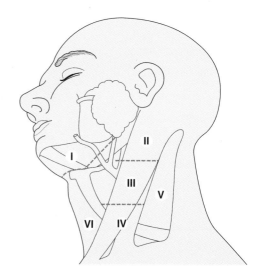

Fig. 16.2 Sloan–Kettering classification of regions of the neck. The hyoid bone and omohyoid muscle are the boundaries between levels II and III, and levels III and IV, respectively.

If there is a lump in the thyroid region, the patient should be given a drink and asked to swallow while the lump is palpated. Movement on swallowing is diagnostic. Laryngeal crepitus can be a useful sign. The larynx is pressed firmly but gently against the cervical spine and moved laterally. A peculiar grating noise should be heard in the normal person. The absence of crepitus suggests a swelling of the soft tissues lying between the cervical spine and the larynx (for example, a pyriform fossa tumour).

Examination of the neck should always include the parotid glands. Any lump should be subjected to the usual routine of inspection, palpation and auscultation and should be accurately measured.

> **Key points**
>
> ➤ A sound understanding of neck anatomy is essential for accurate diagnosis and management.
> ➤ The lymph nodes of the neck are grouped into six levels for staging and prognostic purposes.
> ➤ Examination should be performed in a systematic manner.

Anatomy and examination of the neck

Examination and assessment of the upper aerodigestive tract

The aim of this chapter is to describe a systematic protocol for the examination and assessment of the upper aerodigestive tract. It is particularly applicable when assessing a potentially malignant neck lump. It is however good practice to perform a complete otorhinolaryngological examination on most new patients attending an ENT clinic, because incidental findings of relevance may be discovered and can be treated promptly. A description of the technique of fibreoptic nasopharyngoscopy will be given, followed by a protocol for assessing a patient with a neck lump. Detailed descriptions of the examination of the oral cavity and the larynx are given in Chapters 21 and 25, respectively.

TECHNIQUE OF FLEXIBLE NASOPHARYNGOSCOPY

The flexible nasopharyngoscope most commonly used in the ENT clinic is a fine paediatric instrument. Larger bore instruments with a suction channel and biopsy port are useful in selected cases for more detailed examination and biopsy. Excellent views of the nasal cavity, nasopharynx, oropharynx, upper hypopharynx and larynx can be obtained. The nasal and nasopharyngeal examinations are performed equally well using a rigid 2.7 mm nasal endoscope. A camera attachment, with a monitor and video recording facility, is a useful addition.

The patient is prepared by anaesthetising the nasal cavities and oropharynx with a suitable topical local anaesthetic in conjuction with decongestant. The examiner sits opposite the patient and passes the nasopharyngoscope along the floor of the nasal cavity under direct vision to the nasopharynx, where both eustachian tube orifices, the fossae of Rosenmuller and roof of the nasopharynx are inspected. Once this has been done the patient is asked to breathe through the nose to facilitate passage of the instrument into the oropharynx. If the view through the endoscope becomes obscured by mucus, touching the tip against mucosa or asking the patient to swallow usually clears the end satisfactorily.

The tongue base and valleculae are carefully inspected for abnormalities such as cysts, asymmetry of the tongue base or mucosal lesions. The hypopharynx is inspected for masses and asymmetry. Pooling of saliva in one or both pyriform fossae is a useful sign of an obstructing lesion lower in the pharynx, beyond a point that can be visualised.

Finally, the larynx is inspected (Ch. 25). Fibreoptic examination should be used in conjunction with mirror examination, as the two are complementary: fibreoptic examination is particularly useful in patients with a pronounced gag reflex or an overhanging epiglottis, when the entire length of the vocal cords can be assessed. Video recording of the vocal cord movements is very important in the management of patients with voice disorders.

DIFFERENTIAL DIAGNOSIS OF NECK LUMPS

A useful classification of the differential diagnoses of neck lumps is based on the patient's age. A good history and examination is essential in arriving at a diagnosis. In each age group the approximate order of frequency of diagnosis is shown below:

- Children
  - Infective lymphadenopathy
  - Tuberculosis (including atypical varieties)

- Congenital causes, e.g. haemangioma
- Neoplasms
● Adolescents/young adults
  - Infective lymphadenopathy
  - Branchial and thyroglossal cysts
  - Sialadenitis and salivary gland neoplasms
  - Lymphoma
  - Metastatic papillary thyroid carcinoma
  - Tuberculosis (including atypical varieties)
  - Metastatic squamous cell carcinoma
● Middle-aged/elderly adults
  - Metastatic squamous cell carcinoma
  - Lymphoma
  - Salivary gland neoplasms
  - Infective lymphadenopathy
  - Tuberculosis
  - Other metastatic carcinoma, including thyroid.

THE OCCULT PRIMARY

When a middle-aged or elderly patient presents with a lump in the neck, it must be presumed to be a metastatic squamous cell carcinoma from a primary in the upper aerodigestive tract until proven otherwise. It is a basic oncological principle to find and treat a primary at the same time as a metastasis. Inappropriate investigation and management of the neck node will compromise further management of the primary and may make the prognosis significantly worse. Definitive treatment of the primary may be delayed and made more difficult by incorrectly incising or excising the neck node.

Metastatic squamous cell carcinoma is more likely in the presence of any of the following symptoms: hoarseness, dysphagia, sore throat, otalgia (referred), oral ulceration or haemoptysis. A history of smoking or heavy alcohol intake is significant.

A primary carcinoma may be easily identified on examination. However, the lump may be the sole presenting feature of head and neck cancer; nasopharyngeal carcinoma presents with a neck lump in 60% of cases. The common occult primary sites presenting with a metastatic neck node are shown in the Box 17.1.

■ **Box 17.1**

Metastatic neck nodes: occult primary sites

■ Nasopharynx
■ Tonsil and tongue base
■ Thyroid gland
■ Supraglottic larynx
■ Oral cavity
■ Pyriform fossa
■ Distant sites
  - Bronchus
  - Oesophagus
  - Breast
  - Stomach

The site of the node will give an indication of the site of the primary in many instances (Fig. 17.1).

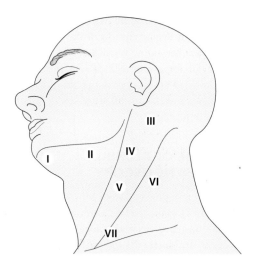

I, II cancer of anterior floor of mouth, lip, anterior two-thirds of tongue, gums and mucosa of cheek

III carcinoma of oropharynx, larynx and Nasopharynx

IV carcinoma of larynx, hypopharynx, nasopharynx, oral cavity

V carcinoma of larynx and hypopharynx, thyroid

VI carcinoma of nasopharynx and skin

VII carcinoma of thyroid, pharynx, upper oesophagus, primary below clavicle

Fig. 17.1 The location of metastatic lymph nodes may be indicative of the primary site.

SYSTEMATIC INVESTIGATION OF A PRESUMED METASTATIC NECK LUMP

In patients with a neck lump presumed to be metastatic squamous cell carcinoma, the following steps should be taken. In one-third a primary will be found in the clinic, in another third a primary will be identified from histological examination, and in another third the primary will be identified on subsequent investigation, or never at all. Systematic investigation comprises:

1. A full history, concentrating on the symptoms and risk factors mentioned above
2. A thorough otorhinolaryngological examination, to include the following:
   - oral cavity, especially
     - the tonsillolingual sulcus
     - the retromolar trigone ('coffin corner')
   - indirect laryngoscopy
   - fibreoptic examination of the upper aerodigestive tract
   - otological examination (nasopharyngeal carcinoma may present with middle ear effusion)
   - systematic neck examination
3. Chest X-ray
4. Other investigations that may be thought necessary; for example, a barium swallow (if there is dysphagia or a low neck node) or haematological investigations
5. Fine-needle aspiration cytology (FNAC) (Box 17.2). This is a reliable test in squamous cell carcinoma and useful in the diagnosis and management of lymphomas and thyroid and salivary gland tumours. If the lesion is cystic, material should be sent both for cytological and microbiological investigation. In such cases a residual lump is suspicious, as is reaccumulation of fluid, and investigations should proceed as described below.

Depending upon the results of these investigations, the patient should be admitted for a panendoscopy. FNAC should be repeated if the first result was inconclusive. If there is an obvious primary, it should be biopsied.

A panendoscopy usually includes the following procedures:

- examination under anaesthetic (EUA) of the oral cavity
- microlaryngoscopy
- pharyngo-oesophagoscopy
- nasopharyngeal examination
- bronchoscopy.

If no primary site is identified, biopsies are taken of the nasopharynx, tongue base and pyriform fossa and a unilateral tonsillectomy is performed.

If lymphoma is the most likely diagnosis on clinical or cytological grounds, the lump should be excised through an incision that can itself be excised and incorporated into a radical neck dissection if the histology in fact turns out to be squamous cell carcinoma. Rarely, once exhaustive investigations have proved to be inconclusive, an incisional or excisional biopsy through a similar incision is necessary to obtain sufficient material for histological diagnosis of other disorders.

Once the initial investigations are complete and a diagnosis made, further radiological investigations such as CT or MRI may be necessary. The patient's treatment plan should then be discussed in a desig-

---

■ Box 17.2

Technique of FNAC

1. Prepare the skin with an alcohol-soaked swab
2. Use a 5 ml or 10 ml syringe and a 22G needle. The syringe may be loaded into a specially designed mount
3. Insert the needle well into the lesion
4. Keeping constant suction on the syringe, make several passes into the lump to aspirate tissue into the needle. Try to avoid aspirating blood (easier said than done!)
5. Remove the needle without suction
6. Smear the tissue thinly on to glass slides. Fixative may be used on the slides (ask advice from your cytologist)
7. Check for haemostasis

Examination and assessment of the upper aerodigestive tract

nated head and neck oncology clinic with other specialists. This would usually include a radiation oncologist, a maxillofacial surgeon, a plastic surgeon, palliative care physicians and nurses, speech therapists and any other interested specialists. Appropriate management of an often complex problem can then be planned to achieve optimum success for a particular patient.

> **Key points**

> ➤ Fibreoptic nasopharyngoscopy is essential in the investigation of most disorders of the pharynx or larynx.
> ➤ Neck nodes are more likely to be malignant with increasing patient age.
> ➤ Investigation of a potentially malignant lymph node should commence with a search for a primary site.
> ➤ A systematic protocol based upon that described in this chapter should be followed in the assessment of a potentially malignant neck node.

Neck swellings

18

A sound knowledge of the anatomy of the neck is, as previously indicated, important in the diagnosis of neck lumps. Of equal importance are the patient's history and clinical examination. Is the swelling midline or is it lateral? If lateral, is it unilateral or are there bilateral swellings? As in most otolaryngological diseases, unilateral symptoms and signs should be viewed with suspicion, especially if of recent onset. Is the swelling tender and acute or painless and chronic? Is there any associated acute or chronic inflammation of the skin of the neck, face or scalp, or of the nose, mouth, pharynx or larynx? Are there any systemic symptoms such as malaise, weight loss or night sweats? If there are multiple lumps they are likely to be enlarged lymph nodes.

Appropriate investigations to confirm the suspected clinical diagnosis should be performed: a full blood count should be routine. If infectious mononucleosis is suspected a monospot test is also performed. In all cases of chronic neck swellings a chest X-ray is requested. Fine-needle aspiration cytology (FNAC) is especially useful in the management of chronic neck lumps. The technique is described in Chapter 17. Cystic fluid may be aspirated and the lump may disappear, which is generally a reassuring sign, although fluid should be sent for analysis and the patient carefully followed up. If the services of a good cytologist are available, a confident diagnosis can often be made, especially in cases of squamous cell carcinoma, and usually in lymphoma and salivary gland neoplasms. Open biopsy should only be carried out with extreme caution, particularly if carcinoma is suspected. Excisional biopsy should be the treatment of choice, although an incisional biopsy may be necessary in large lesions of unknown aetiology that are adherent to vital structures. Any incision in the neck should be planned so that it can be incorporated into a subsequent neck dissection incision if necessary.

CONGENITAL CERVICAL SWELLINGS AND FISTULAE

Thyroglossal cyst or fistula

A thyroglossal cyst usually presents in childhood as a midline infrahyoid swelling (Fig. 18.1). It is a cystic space in the thyroglossal tract, the remnant of the embryological migration of the thyroid gland from the foramen caecum at the base of the tongue to

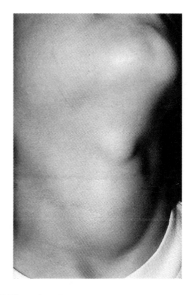

Fig. 18.1 Thyroglossal cyst.

137

the root of the neck along the thyroglossal duct. The cyst can occur at any level along this route. The cyst moves on swallowing because it is attached to the thyroid gland, and also on protruding the tongue because of its attachment to this structure.

A thyroglossal cyst may become infected, forming an abscess which then discharges through the skin of the neck. The discharge may continue despite treatment, forming a fistula.

Surgical management should be preceded by an ultrasound examination of the neck to ensure that there is a normal thyroid gland. Sistrunk's procedure, in which the cyst or fistula is excised together with the thyroglossal tract up to the base of the tongue and the central portion of the hyoid bone, minimises the chance of recurrence.

Branchial sinuses and fistulae

These are the result of anomalies of development of the branchial arches. Initially there are six arches but the fifth is transient. Between the remaining five mesodermal arches there are four branchial pouches lined with endoderm and four branchial grooves lined with ectoderm. These pouches and grooves are separated by a thin layer of mesoderm (Fig. 18.2). A variety of anomalies are recognised: an ectodermal or endodermal pouch may persist as a

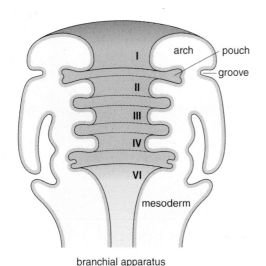

Fig. 18.2 Coronal cross-section through embryonic throat.

branchial sinus; the mesodermal layer may break down, resulting in a branchial fistula; or a branchial cyst can occur if part of a branchial groove or pouch becomes separated from the surface and fails to resorb. Lesions are occasionally bilateral and there may be a positive family history.

Theoretically a first arch fistula would extend from the skin of the neck, between the internal and external carotid arteries to the region of the eustachian tube orifice, and a second arch fistula from the skin of the lower third of the neck anterior to the sternocleidomastoid muscle, between the internal and external carotid arteries to the supratonsillar fossa. Third and fourth arch fistulae open at a similar site on the neck, the former passing between the common carotid artery and the vagus nerve to the pyriform fossa, and the latter caudal to the arch of the aorta or the right subclavian artery to the upper oesophagus or pyriform fossa. Second arch fistulae are the most common. A collaural fistula extends from the external auditory meatus to the neck, emerging above the hyoid between the angle of the mandible and the sternocleidomastoid muscle; it runs through the parotid gland and has a variable relation to the facial nerve. It is caused by persistence of the ventral part of the first branchial groove.

Branchial apparatus anomalies may present with cutaneous pits or skin tags; persistent mucous discharge may be a feature and recurrent infection and abscess formation are common complications. Treatment is by complete excision, taking care to avoid damage to adjacent structures.

Cervical dermoid

Dermoid cysts and sinuses can occur in the neck and are usually found above the hyoid bone in the midline. They should be excised if symptomatic.

Cystic hygroma

This is a hamartomatous malformation of the lymphatic system. Multilocular masses with thin walls enclose straw-coloured fluid. Extensive cervicofacial swelling is present at birth (Fig. 18.3) and may be so large as to compromise the airway, necessitating tracheostomy. The lesion is usually slow-growing

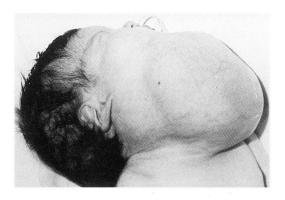

Fig. 18.3 Huge cystic hygroma.

unless there is internal venous haemorrhage or infective lymphangitis. Underlying hypertrophy of the maxilla and mandible may develop. Resection is usually indicated both for functional and for cosmetic improvement. Normal structures such as the facial nerve are at risk in this surgery because there is an absence of the usual tissue planes. Encouraging results have been reported with intralesional OK-432, an immunomodulatory agent prepared from an attenuated strain of *Streptococcus pyogenes*, which has a sclerosing effect.

ACQUIRED SWELLINGS

The common causes of acquired swellings in the neck can be considered in the following categories:

- Neck space infections
  - Ludwig's angina
  - Submandibular abscess
  - Retropharyngeal and parapharyngeal abscess
- Lymphadenopathy
  - Acute infections
    Viral (Infectious mononucleosis)
    Bacterial
  - Chronic infections
    Tuberculosis
    HIV
    Toxoplasmosis
    Cat scratch disease
    Actinomycosis
    Brucellosis

- Inflammatory
  - Sarcoidosis
- Neoplastic
  - Lymphoma
  - Metastatic carcinoma
    Squamous carcinoma from head and neck primary
    Thyroid carcinoma
    Adenocarcinoma from distant primary
- Branchial cyst
- Vascular
  - Carotid body tumour
- Neurological
  - Schwannoma
  - Neurilemmoma
- Thyroid lesions
- Salivary gland lesions.

ACUTE INFECTIONS

Acute lymphadenitis

This is the most frequent cause of neck swellings. The lymphadenopathy is reactive to an acute infection of the mouth, tonsils (most commonly) or pharynx. Dental sepsis is another well-known cause. An infection of the skin of the face or scalp may lead to lymphadenopathy in the draining nodes. In acute tonsillitis the lymphadenopathy is acute in onset, tender and bilateral. The involved nodes are the jugulodigastric nodes, and resolution of the lymphadenopathy follows resolution of the illness. If the diagnosis is infectious mononucleosis, the lymphadenopathy may be massive and more persistent. Treatment is directed at the underlying cause. Suppuration and development of a cervical abscess is rare but may occur after a prolonged illness and will usually be unilateral. Diagnosis is clinical (but may be supported by ultrasonography) and treatment is by incision and drainage.

Infectious mononucleosis

Patients usually have fever, sore throat and lymphadenopathy (often massive). There may be a rash, which is common if amoxycillin has been administered. More serious complications include haematological abnormalities, impaired liver function, splenic rupture, encephalitis and cranial nerve palsies. On examination the tonsils are often considerably enlarged, with a diagnostic plaque covering them. Petechial haemorrhages may be present on the soft palate. Tonsillar enlargement may be so great that they meet in the midline and cause stertor. Treatment is supportive.

Ludwig's angina

This is an acute cellulitis of the submandibular triangle deep to the mylohyoid muscle. It usually arises from sepsis in the oral cavity (including teeth) or pharynx which reaches the tissues of the neck directly.

Infection is limited by the attachment of the deep cervical fascia to the mandible and hyoid bone so that tension rises, making pain a prominent feature. The infection tracks posteriorly in the deep spaces; laryngeal oedema is a dangerous complication. The

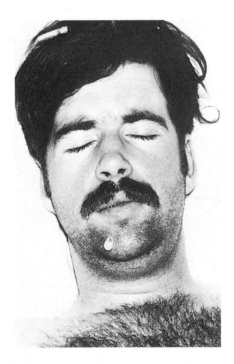

Fig. 18.4 Ludwig's angina. Note the brawny neck swelling, the ill appearance of the patient and the saliva drooling from the mouth.

patient is ill and toxic with an indurated swelling of the submandibular triangle. There is oedema of the floor of the mouth, with the tongue pushed upwards (Fig. 18.4).

Aggressive treatment with intravenous antibiotics to cover anaerobes may control the infection in the early stages; incision and drainage are otherwise necessary, incising all fascial planes widely to release the tension on the infected areas. Endotracheal intubation or a tracheostomy may be necessary to protect the airway.

Retropharyngeal and parapharyngeal abscesses

Infection, usually arising from a suppurating lymph node, may develop in the deep neck spaces, which are bounded by dense, well-defined fascia. Parapharyngeal (or lateral pharyngeal) space infection develops as a result of acute tonsillitis (or a peritonsillar abscess) or dental infection. It may point laterally in the neck but fluctuation may be absent because the infection is so deep. Retropharyngeal abscesses are most commonly the result of a suppurating retropharyngeal node but may be secondary to a penetrating injury of the pharynx, or more rarely secondary to tuberculosis of the cervical spine. Infections of the retropharyngeal space can track down into the chest, causing mediastinitis.

Such patients are usually severely ill with a high pyrexia and possibly dehydrated. They will complain of dysphagia and pain in the neck and may have stridor because of laryngeal oedema. A brawny, diffuse, tender swelling is often present and the neck may be thickened. Laryngeal crepitus may be absent. A full blood count and estimation of urea and electrolytes and blood glucose should be performed (the patient may be immunocompromised because of diabetes) and the patient resuscitated. The state of the airway should govern definitive management. A lateral soft tissue neck radiograph may be diagnostic of a retropharyngeal abscess (Fig. 18.5A) and CT can be invaluable in locating an abscess cavity (Fig. 18.5B). While conservative management with intravenous antibiotics may be appropriate in selected cases, these patients usually require external surgical drainage; wide exposure of the affected neck spaces is essential and large drains are inserted.

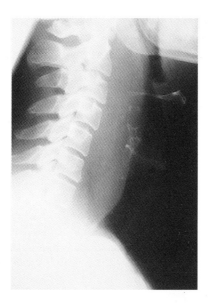

(a)

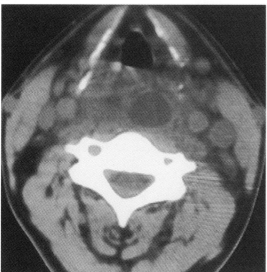

(b)

Fig. 18.5 Patient with retropharyngeal abscess. (a) Plain lateral neck radiograph with marked swelling of the prevertebral soft tissues. (b) Axial CT scan. Abscess cavity seen as lucent area within swollen prevertebral soft tissues.

If the airway is at risk, endotracheal intubation or tracheostomy (extremely difficult in such cases) may be necessary.

CHRONIC INFECTIONS

Tuberculosis

Tuberculosis may present in the neck as a chronic painless enlarged lymph node. There can be associated erythema of the skin, and occasionally a chronically discharging sinus. The nodes involved can be multiple. While tuberculosis occurs more commonly in those from the Indian subcontinent and in immunocompromised patients, mycobacterial lymphadenitis can occur in healthy individuals as the only presenting symptom. Atypical mycobacteria (such as *Mycobacterium avium*) account for the majority of cases in most series from more developed countries. These bacteria are resistant to the usual antituberculous treatment. Investigation of a suspected tuberculous node should include a good history for contact tracing, a chest radiograph, a Mantoux test (although this is often confusing) and FNAC, which may yield alcohol – and acid-fast bacilli. Management of the tuberculous node is by complete excision, which obviates the need for prolonged chemotherapy and has a low incidence of persistent infection in the form of skin sinuses (Fig. 18.6).

HIV infection

Otolaryngological involvement in AIDS is common and cervical lymphadenopathy may be part of the persistent generalised lymphadenopathy (PGL) complex. The diagnosis is usually known prior to the patient developing multiple lymphadenopathy and there is rarely a place for diagnostic biopsy of a cervical node.

BRANCHIAL CYSTS

These acquired swellings of the neck are most common in young adults. Their pathogenesis has been hotly debated and it is most likely that they arise from secretion of fluid from epithelial tissue included within a cervical lymph node, although occasionally a tract can be found extending between the carotid arteries to the tonsil, suggesting a second branchial arch origin (see above).

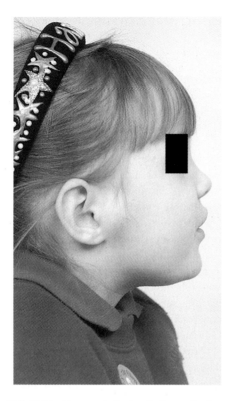

Fig. 18.6 Child with preauricular lymphadenopathy due to an atypical mycobacterium.

Branchial cysts are single and globular, lying in the upper part of the anterior triangle closely applied to the anterior aspect of sternomastoid. Diagnosis is clinical, helped by FNAC (the fluid should always be sent for cytological examination). Excision is recommended to prevent infection and for histological purposes; the differential diagnoses include metastatic papillary carcinoma of the thyroid, lymphoma (Fig. 18.7) and carotid body tumour.

BENIGN TUMOURS

Carotid body tumour

Tumours of the carotid body (chemodectomas) are extremely rare but pose a diagnostic challenge. They arise in a similar site and in a similar age group to branchial cysts but are hard and said to be mobile only in the transverse plane, as they are attached to the carotid artery, preventing movement in a craniocaudal direction. Needle aspiration is safe because of the small size of vessels in the tumour but the aspirate will yield bloody fluid and the lesion will not disappear. Diagnosis can be suspected on ultrasonography or CT and confirmed on MRI and angiography. It is prudent for this reason to perform an ultrasound or CT scan on all deep neck lumps in this area. Chemodectomas may be multiple in the neck or elsewhere (especially if there is a family history) and are associated with phaeochromocytomas.

Treatment is by excision, performed in conjunction with a vascular surgeon. If a lump is explored and a carotid body tumour discovered inadvertently, the wound should be closed and further investigations carried out prior to formal excision.

Neurogenic tumours

Vagal schwannomas and neurilemmomas are rare but present as a slowly enlarging lump in the upper part of the neck. There may be associated symptoms of hoarseness (if there is a palsy of the vagus nerve) and also intracranial signs if there is extension into the skull base. Detailed imaging of the skull base is required and surgical excision should be undertaken by a surgeon experienced in skull-base procedures.

LYMPHOMAS

A neck lump may be the presenting feature of Hodgkin's or non-Hodgkin's lymphoma. This is a disease of young and middle-aged adults and characteristically presents with one or more bean-sized rubbery nodes in the neck which may wax and wane in size but are generally slow growing. Careful examination of other lymph node groups in the body as well as the liver and spleen is essential as is a chest radiograph. Systemic symptoms such as night sweats and weight loss indicate a poorer prognosis. Excision biopsy is necessary for diagnosis and the unfixed node should usually be sent to the laboratory for analysis.

Treatment depends upon the staging (which is assessed according to standard protocols) and is undertaken by a specialist in lymphoma management.

If the disease is localised to the neck radiotherapy is the preferred option, whereas, if it is widespread combination chemotherapy may be given (Fig. 18.7).

METASTATIC LYMPHADENOPATHY

It is good clinical practice to suspect that a lump in the neck is malignant until proved otherwise (Fig. 18.7). This is especially true in the older patient with a hard lump with associated symptoms, as discussed in Chapter 17. The most common pathology is a primary squamous cell carcinoma arising in the upper aerodigestive tract. Much more rarely, pathological examination indicates metastatic thyroid carcinoma or adenocarcinoma arising from the bronchus, stomach or breast. FNAC is helpful in making the pathological diagnosis at the same time as a complete upper aerodigestive tract examination is carried out. The neck node should be treated in conjunction with the primary, not in isolation.

The prognosis of head and neck cancer is profoundly affected by the presence of metastatic lymphadenopathy and is related to the site, size and number of involved nodes and whether there is any extracapsular spread of disease. Neck disease should be carefully staged according to the Tumour, Node, Metastasis (TNM) classification (Box 18.1) and the level recorded according to Figure 16.2. It should be noted that this is a clinical classification and a patient with a head and neck primary but no palpable lymph nodes may still have occult lymphatic metastases, a situation more common in some tumours (for example, hypopharyngeal tumours) than others.

■ Box 18.1

Staging of regional lymph nodes in head and neck cancer

- N0 No regional lymph node metastasis palpable
- N1 Metastasis palpable in a single ipsilateral lymph node. 3 cm or less in greatest dimension
- N2a Metastasis in a single ipsilateral node, more than 3 cm but not more than 6 cm in greatest dimension
- N2b Metastasis in multiple ipsilateral nodes, none more than 6 cm in greatest dimension
- N2c Metastasis in bilateral or contralateral nodes, none more than 6 cm in greatest dimension
- N3 Metastasis in any lymph node more than 6 cm in greatest dimension

---

The management of metastatic lymphadenopathy is generally surgical, with adjuvant postoperative radiotherapy in selected cases. Primary radiotherapy has less curative effect on larger tumour masses than smaller ones but it has a role in the palliation of nodal disease that is deemed incurable by surgery.

Metastatic lymphadenopathy of the neck should be treated surgically by a systematic dissection of the neck nodes and other structures. A radical neck dissection involves clearance of all lymph nodes, the internal jugular vein, the spinal accessory nerve and the submandibular salivary gland. In certain cases

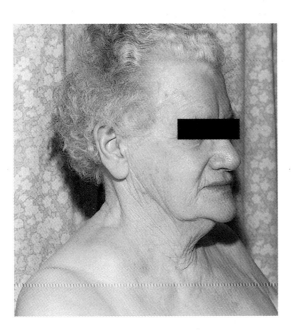

Fig. 18.7 Lymphoma presenting as a lump in the posterior triangle of the neck.

the dissection can be more selective without compromising oncological principles, thus preserving function and quality of life to a greater extent.

THYROID LESIONS

See Chapter 19.

SALIVARY GLAND LESIONS

See Chapter 23.

> **Key points**
>
> ➤ A good knowledge of anatomy combined with history and examination will usually give a firm indication of the diagnosis of a neck swelling.
> ➤ Multiple lumps are almost invariably lymph nodes.
> ➤ Neck space infections may be deep and difficult to diagnose clinically but can lead to serious complications.
> ➤ Fine-needle aspiration cytology (FNAC) is a very useful diagnostic tool for benign and malignant lumps.
> ➤ Malignant lumps should be staged accurately and managed in conjunction with the primary.

Thyroid

ANATOMY

The thyroid gland is an endocrine gland situated in the root of the neck. It is a bilobed structure, the lobes being connected by an isthmus. A pyramidal lobe may extend superiorly from the isthmus, reminding one of the more cranial embryological origin of the gland. Each lobe and the isthmus is attached to the trachea by the ligament of Berry, which explains why the gland and any lumps within it move on swallowing. The gland is surrounded by the pretracheal fascia and is covered anteriorly by the strap muscles (sternohyoid and sternothyroid muscles).

The posterior relations of the thyroid lobe are of crucial importance. The recurrent laryngeal nerve runs up the tracheo-oesophageal groove to pass behind the cricothyroid joint. Because it is in intimate relationship with the inferior thyroid artery, the nerve must to be positively identified before the artery is divided. The external laryngeal nerve runs close to the superior thyroid artery and division of that artery has to be as close as possible with the superior lobe of the thyroid to avoid damage; division of this nerve leads to more subtle changes in the voice than division of the recurrent nerve and may only be noticeable in those who use their voice professionally.

A superior and inferior parathyroid gland lie on the posterior aspect of the thyroid lobe; they are pale yellow pea-sized structures that secrete parathyroid hormone involved in calcium metabolism.

PHYSIOLOGY

The thyroid gland contains many follicles into which thyroxine (T_4) is secreted. Production of this hormone is regulated by the influence of thyroid-stimulating hormone (TSH) produced by the hypothalamic–pituitary axis under the influence of thyrotrophin–releasing hormone (TRH). T_4 is protein bound to a large extent in the bloodstream and converted peripherally into tri-iodothyronine (T_3) which is more active than T_4. The thyroid hormones play an important part in the regulation of metabolism, and the levels within the bloodstream influence the production of TSH in a negative-feedback manner.

INVESTIGATION OF THE THYROID LUMP

Thyroid function tests

Estimation of the levels of T_3 and T_4 will provide evidence of the thyroid status (euthyroid, hypothyroid or hyperthyroid), while TSH levels will assess whether the normal homeostatic mechanisms are functioning correctly. In well-differentiated thyroid cancer, TSH levels are suppressed by therapy with T_3 or T_4 because high levels of TSH stimulate tumour growth.

Thyroid

Imaging

Ultrasonography

Ultrasound examination is useful in assessing thyroid lumps. It will confirm whether a lump is cystic or solid and whether it is single or solitary, which has significance in the management of thyroid masses.

Radioisotope scanning

This imaging technique is used in the investigation of the function of solitary nodules. The most commonly used isotope is technetium-99. A 'cold' nodule against a normally functioning gland suggests a non-functioning nodule (suspicious of malignancy), while a 'hot' nodule against a suppressed gland suggests an autonomously functioning nodule, suppressing normal hormone production. Iodine-131 scans are useful in following up disease after total thyroidectomy for well-differentiated thyroid cancer.

Computerised tomography

CT is useful in investigating retrosternal extension and compression or deviation of the trachea, as well as in assessing the nodal status or invasion of surrounding structures. It does not need to be used routinely in the investigation of thyroid lumps.

Fine-needle aspiration cytology

If there is an experienced cytologist available, FNAC can be very useful in assessing the nature of a thyroid lump. This test distinguishes between papillary and follicular lesions as well as the rarer forms of tumour (including lymphoma) but cannot be used to comment on the presence of malignancy in follicular lesions because this relies upon the presence of vascular and extracapsular invasion. Open biopsy is rarely necessary.

MANAGEMENT OF THE THYROID LUMP

The management of a patient presenting with a solitary mass in the thyroid is aimed at identifying potentially malignant lumps. Careful examination may identify several lumps of different size consistent with a multinodular goitre and patients can be safely reassured of the benign nature of this condition. Aspiration of one of the nodules usually produces cystic fluid containing abundant colloid material. A multinodular goitre is often treated by lobectomy or subtotal thyroidectomy because of the risk of tracheal compression.

A clinically solitary lump should be investigated by FNAC and ultrasonography. The ultrasound may reveal this to be a dominant nodule in a multinodular goitre, in which case the patient can be reassured. The FNAC may produce cystic fluid, or – if solid – cellular material, which can be very helpful in diagnosis. The cells may be papillary; these are large cells with abundant cytoplasm and prominent nuclei ('Orphan Annie' cells) and the cytologist can estimate the degree of malignancy. If the cells are follicular malignancy cannot be estimated because follicular carcinoma is differentiated from adenoma on the basis of the degree of vascular and extracapsular invasion.

Some clinicians will carry out a radioisotope scan. 'Cold' nodules suggest malignancy; 'hot' nodules do not.

These investigations help in planning the correct management. It would be rare for a solitary thyroid nodule not to be removed surgically, even if thought to be benign, but the extent of resection is governed by the results of investigations. Sometimes investigations prove to be unhelpful, in which case lobectomy is carried out to excise the whole lump for diagnosis, with further definitive surgery if necessary.

THYROID NEOPLASMS

Box 19.1 lists the classification of thyroid neoplasms. Thyroid cancer is uncommon but increasing in incidence. Most cases present between the ages of 25 and 65. Important predisposing factors include radiation to the neck in infancy and childhood for benign conditions such as acne or thymus enlargement.

Papillary and follicular carcinoma are known as well-differentiated carcinomas and are most common in young adults, more commonly females. Papillary carcinoma is often multicentric and growth is partially under the influence of TSH.

■ Box 19.1

Classification of thyroid neoplasms

- Adenoma
  - Papillary
  - Follicular
- Carcinoma
  - Papillary
  - Follicular
  - Medullary
  - Anaplastic
  - Squamous cell
- Lymphoma
- Metastatic tumours

much more aggressive tumours metastasising early and a very poor prognosis. Medullary carcinoma is occasionally familial and associated with the multiple endocrine neoplasia (MEN) syndrome; the patient and family should be screened for this by genetic testing and calcitonin levels. Treatment is by total thyroidectomy. Anaplastic carcinoma frequently presents with airway obstruction, and tracheostomy can be a challenging exercise in such patients. The differential diagnosis is lymphoma and open biopsy is therefore indicated, as the prognosis is so different. The disease may be so advanced at presentation that treatment is symptomatic only. Otherwise it is by total thyroidectomy and adjuvant radiotherapy, or radiotherapy alone as palliative treatment.

Well-differentiated thyroid cancer may present with a metastatic neck node but the survival is not worsened by this occurrence. Indeed, provided there is no extrathyroid spread of the primary or distant metastases, well-differentiated thyroid cancer carries an excellent prognosis, especially in the young adult.

Treatment of papillary carcinoma is by subtotal or total thyroidectomy with a postoperative ablative dose of iodine-131 and suppression of TSH by thyroxine therapy. The more aggressive follicular carcinoma is treated by total thyroidectomy and parathyroid preservation: external beam radiotherapy is used in recurrent disease.

Poorly differentiated (medullary and anaplastic) carcinomas occur in older people and are rare, with

➤ **Key points**

- ➤ Lumps in the thyroid gland move on swallowing.
- ➤ Solitary lumps need to be investigated to exclude malignancy.
- ➤ Ultrasonography and FNAC are the most useful investigations in the management of thyroid lumps.
- ➤ Well-differentiated thyroid cancer has an excellent prognosis, whereas poorly differentiated tumours carry a very poor prognosis.

THE MOUTH AND SALIVARY GLANDS

4

Anatomy and physiology of the mouth and salivary glands

20

While diseases of the oral cavity are usually managed by oral and maxillofacial surgeons, otolaryngologists need to have a basic understanding of these diseases and should be thoroughly conversant with the anatomy and examination of the oral cavity, as the latter should be a routine part of an otolaryngological examination.

ORAL ANATOMY

The oral cavity is that area from the lips to the anterior faucial pillars, so the tonsils are part of the oropharynx. It is lined by stratified squamous epithelium throughout, with numerous taste papillae scattered about, as well as many minor salivary glands that may give rise to tumours generally presenting with a hard, non-ulcerating lump.

The roof of the mouth consists of the hard palate and upper alveolus. This is part of the maxillary bone and constitutes the floor of the nasal cavity and maxillary sinuses, so the upper molar and premolar teeth are closely related to the floor of the sinus. Posteriorly is the curtain-like soft palate which forms the floor of the nasopharynx (Fig. 20.1).

The floor of the mouth consists of a muscular diaphragm slung between the mandible and the hyoid bone, which supports the body of the tongue. The tongue itself is a strong, muscular mobile structure. It is important in normal speech and the first stage of swallowing. The margin between its anterior two-thirds and its posterior one-third (which lies in the oropharynx) is delineated by the large and prominent vallate papillae.

There are about 9000 taste buds in the adult, mainly on the peripheral parts of the dorsum of the tongue and most easily found in the groove sur-rounding the vallate papillae. A few taste buds also occur on the soft palate. There are only four taste sensations: sweet, sour, salt and bitter. Sweetness is mainly perceived on the tip of the tongue, bitter at the root, salt and sour along the edges.

The oral cavity has a large sensory representation in the cerebral cortex. Taste sensation from the anterior two-thirds of the tongue is via the chorda tympani, and via the glossopharyngeal nerve for the posterior one-third. This sensation passes to the nucleus of the tractus solitarius in the brainstem.

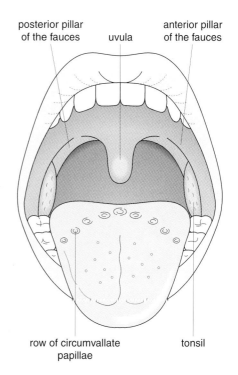

Fig. 20.1 Mouth and oropharynx.

151

Common sensation is via branches of the mandibular nerve, and motor supply of the tongue via the hypoglossal nerve.

The frenulum is a prominent sharp band of mucosa connecting the tongue to the floor of the mouth in the midline. If the attachment is too great the tongue cannot be protruded and 'tongue tie' results. On either side of the frenulum lie the sublingual salivary glands, closely related to the submandibular ducts (Wharton's duct) which run forward from the submandibular gland to open close to the midline, where saliva can be easily expressed.

The buccal cavities lie laterally to the teeth and are bounded by the alveolar margins and the mobile facial muscles (buccinator) as well as the masseter muscle. The parotid duct (Stensen's duct) enters the mouth in the buccal cavity opposite the second upper molar tooth.

DENTITION

There are two generations of teeth in humans: the deciduous and permanent dentitions. Permanent dentition starts to replace the deciduous teeth in a set pattern from the 6th year. The full adult dentition consists of 32 teeth, with two incisors, one canine, two premolar and three molar teeth in each quadrant. The quadrants are derived from an imaginary cross imposed when looking at the subject (Fig. 20.2). Well-recognised symbols describe the teeth according to their quadrants. Thus the maxillary left first molar is designated |6 .

SALIVARY GLANDS

There are three paired major salivary glands: the parotid, submandibular and sublingual glands. Embryologically they are derived from epithelium of the oral cavity. The salivary glands produce more than 1 litre of saliva each day, some of it in response to food stimuli and some continuously. Each gland produces saliva of different consistencies – the parotid producing serous saliva and the submandibular gland more mucous fluid. Saliva lubricates the mouth, helping to prevent infection, and starts the digestive process in the mouth. Loss of saliva production (xerostomia) is a disabling condition that follows radiotherapy to the oral cavity and salivary glands, as well as occurring in Sjögren's syndrome.

The parotid gland overlies the lateral part of the face and upper neck (Fig. 21.1). It has a large superficial lobe, and a smaller deep lobe lying deep to the mandible in the parapharyngeal space. Tumours of the deep lobe can present as pharyngeal swellings. The most important relation of the gland is the facial nerve, which passes into the gland immediately it leaves the stylomastoid foramen, and divides into its terminal branches within the gland. It is at risk during parotid surgery. The gland is impalpable in the normal subject.

The submandibular gland is a walnut-sized gland that lies in the submandibular triangle deep to the platysma and cervical fascia. This fascia is tightly bound to the hyoid bone and mandible, so any swelling of the gland causes considerable pain. The

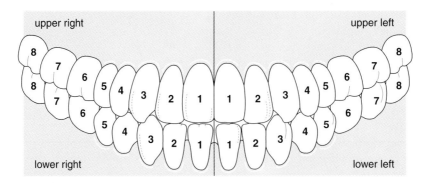

Fig. 20.2 The standard system for designating permanent teeth. The appropriate quadrant is indicated by two perpendicular lines, the point at which they join indicating the midpoint in both horizontal and vertical planes. Thus 6| = upper right 6.

normal gland is palpable in thin patients. It has a superficial lobe that is partially covered by the mandible, which it indents, and a deep lobe that lies deep to the mylohyoid muscle within the mouth. The submandibular duct runs forward from the deep lobe in a tortuous course to the papilla centrally. During its course it twice crosses the lingual nerve, which is thus at risk in operations to remove stones from the duct. The submandibular branch of the facial nerve lies superficial to the deep cervical fascia over the gland and is at risk of damage if a surgical incision is placed too high.

Examination and assessment of the mouth and salivary glands

21

ORAL CAVITY

Examination of the oral cavity has to be carried out in a thorough and systematic manner; there are many nooks and crannies in the mouth where disease can easily be missed if they are not inspected. It is from bitter experience that the tonsillolingual sulcus is otherwise known as 'coffin corner', where tumours are missed until too far advanced.

The first golden rule is always to remove the dentures if the patient is edentulous. These should be inspected for infection or rough areas that may be causing ulceration in corresponding areas of the mucosa. The mouth is best examined using a head light and two tongue spatulae. The buccal cavities and gingival sulci are first inspected, then the teeth for signs of caries and periodontal disease. The patient is then asked to touch the roof of the mouth with the tongue so that the floor of the mouth can be examined and lastly the tonsillolingual sulci and dorsum of the tongue. This should be followed by bimanual palpation of the floor of the mouth (looking in particular for stones in the submandibular ducts) and palpation of the masseter muscle from within the mouth. Movements of the tongue and jaw should be noted (and any trismus excluded) and the temporomandibular joint carefully examined, feeling for limitation of the range of movement and crepitus indicating arthritis of the joint.

SALIVARY GLANDS

The submandibular gland needs to be scrutinised both externally – standing behind the patient – and bimanually. Lesions of the submandibular triangle that are within the gland are more likely to be palpable from within the mouth than, for example, submandibular lymphadenopathy. As mentioned above, the ducts need to be palpated to exclude calculi.

The parotid gland is only palpable if abnormal. A lump in the parotid region is assumed to be a lesion of the parotid until proven otherwise. Enlargements of the parotid will either be generalised swellings of the whole gland, such as in parotitis, or localised lesions, for example a pleomorphic adenoma (Fig. 21.1).

Examination of the oral cavity and salivary glands should be followed by a careful examination of the neck.

INVESTIGATIONS

Plain radiography is still used extensively in the investigation of oral disease. An orthopantomogram (OPG) is a plain radiograph of the whole of the mandible and is very useful in investigating dental

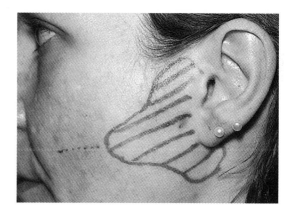

Fig. 21.1 Outline of the parotid gland and duct.

disease, tumour invasion of the mandible and temporomandibular joint dysfunction. Submandibular duct calculi are generally radio-opaque and best seen on an occlusal radiograph. Parotid calculi are usually radiolucent.

Salivary gland disease can be investigated using a number of techniques, depending upon the suspected pathology. Malignant or deep lobe parotid tumours are best imaged using CT or MRI. Sialography will help in the assessment of sialolithiasis, and salivary scintigraphy is useful in the investigation of disordered function, such as in Sjögren's syndrome. Fine needle aspiration cytology is useful in guiding the management of a patient with a suspected tumour if the services of a good cytologist are available.

> **Key points**

> ➤ The oral cavity is a dynamic structure.
> ➤ Oral cavity examination needs to be carried out systematically using a head light and two spatulae.
> ➤ A lump in the parotid region is a tumour of the parotid until proved otherwise.
> ➤ Knowledge of the facial nerve anatomy is crucial in managing salivary gland disease.
> ➤ Plain radiography has an important role to play in the investigation of oral cavity disease.

Oral cavity

22

Because an oral examination is an integral part of a thorough otolaryngological examination, the clinician needs to be aware of common diseases affecting the oral cavity. This chapter gives a brief overview of the more common diseases and how they may interact with otolaryngological disease.

PERIODONTAL DISEASE

Periodontitis is a common disorder, affecting up to 20% of the adult population, where the periodontal ligament (bridging the gap between the bone of the jaw and the tooth and stabilising the tooth in its socket) is destroyed. It is caused by inflammation secondary to bacterial plaque being deposited on the teeth as a result of poor oral hygiene. Smoking and diabetes are the principal exacerbating factors. Unlike the less severe gingivitis, it is irreversible because of the loss of attachment of the tooth.

Clinically patients present with painful, bleeding gums. Examination usually reveals bacterial plaque, as well as resorption of the gingival margin and increased pocketing around the tooth. Periodontal abscesses may result. The microbiology is complex, with a number of organisms, including anaerobes, being implicated. The central event, however, is the destruction of the periodontal attachment by host mechanisms in response to a wide range of organisms.

Treatment is local and topical. Plaque control is the mainstay of treatment, and clear instructions need to be given by a dental hygienist on how to achieve this. The use of dental floss and a 0.2% chlorhexidine mouth rinse twice a day are effective. The principal antibiotics used are the tetracyclines and metronidazole but these must be viewed as an adjunct to topical treatment. Surgical treatment involves debriding diseased tissue so that plaque control can be more easily achieved.

ORAL ULCERATION

Box 22.1 lists the causes of oral ulceration.

Aphthous ulceration

Aphthous ulceration may be major or minor. Minor aphthous ulceration is a very common condition and consists of 'crops' of small, punched out, intensely

---

■ Box 22.1

Causes of oral ulceration

- Mucosal disease
  - Aphthous ulceration
    - major
    - minor
  - Herpetic gingivostomatitis
  - Trauma
    - dentures and sharp teeth
    - thermal trauma
  - Stevens–Johnson syndrome
  - Behçet's disease
  - Chronic specific infection
    - syphilis
    - tuberculosis
  - Pemphigus
    - Benign mucous membrane
  - Pemphigoid
  - Agranulocytosis
  - HIV
- Oral cancer

Oral cavity

painful ulcers on the mucous membrane of the oral cavity. They occur on a recurrent basis and last for about 7–10 days. The aetiology is unknown and in particular an infectious cause has not been proven. An immunological mechanism may be involved. Rarely, they may be associated with a gluten enteropathy. A full blood count should be carried out to identify any rare haematological causes of oral ulceration.

Treatment is symptomatic, with judicious use of pastes, gels and antibiotic mouthwashes to prevent secondary infection. If used at the optimum time (that is, at the very first indication of ulceration), topical steroid creams are effective in aborting progression of the ulcers.

Major aphthous ulceration is a longer lasting problem that is less common than the minor variety. Large ulcers appear on the oral mucosa (commonly the hard palate) and can be very painful. The pathogenesis is as unclear as in the minor aphthae. Treatment is more aggressive; steroid and antibiotic mouthwashes are useful and a short course of systemic steroids may be effective. Any persistent ulcer should be biopsied to exclude malignancy.

Herpetiform ulceration

These ulcers are not necessarily herpetic in origin, although they are similar in appearance to lesions caused by the herpes virus: in appearance, they are small grey lesions that can be missed on examination but cause a disproportionate degree of pain. They are more common in women and the ulcers persist for about 1 week. There is no response to steroid therapy but the use of tetracycline mouthwashes is effective.

Trauma

Persistent irritation of an area of the oral mucosa by ill-fitting dentures or sharp teeth can cause oral ulceration, which may be painful, especially if secondary infections develop. Careful examination of the denture or teeth will reveal if this is the cause. The denture should be adjusted for a comfortable fit. If there is any doubt about the diagnosis a biopsy should be taken to exclude malignancy.

HIV INFECTION

Acquired immune deficiency syndrome (AIDS) is caused by the human immunodeficiency virus (HIV) that specifically attacks the T lymphocytes. Infection may precede development of AIDS by many years. During this time 40% of patients will present with head and neck disease. The degree of immunological impairment can be estimated by measuring the levels of CD4+ and CD8+ T lymphocyte subsets. Oral manifestations of AIDS include:

- *Oral candidiasis.* This is common and caused by immune impairment, and it may affect the pharynx and oesophagus as well as the mouth. Topical treatment with nystatin can be effective but systemic antifungals are often necessary.
- *Herpes virus infection.* Herpes infection is often prolonged in patients with AIDS and may be associated with neurological involvement. Infection with herpes simplex, zoster, cytomegalovirus and Epstein–Barr virus is common.
- *Bacterial infections.* Periodontal disease may be rampant and unusual bacterial infections may occur, for example atypical mycobacterial infections.

LICHEN PLANUS

An associated skin disease is usually seen with this condition. The aetiology is unknown and two variants are described: reticular (or non-erosive) and erosive. The non-erosive type gives rise to raised lesions on the buccal mucosa, often with a bluish tinge. The erosive type presents as erythematous lesions which may be raised and ulcerated. A biopsy is necessary in these cases to exclude leucoplakia and carcinoma. There may be an increased risk of cancer in erosive lichen planus: these cases should be kept under review. Local steroids are useful in the management of the erosive type.

LEUCOPLAKIA

This is diagnosed clinically. White patches on the oral mucosa are abnormal: if they can be removed with a spatula the diagnosis is usually candida. The aetiology of leucoplakia is unknown but there is an increased risk of carcinoma in such patients. Histologically, leucoplakia can be graded from mild atypia to dysplasia and carcinoma in situ. The term erythroplakia is reserved for areas of erythematous change and these areas show a higher propensity for malignancy. Treatment is by excision and this is best performed using the KTP laser.

ORAL CANCER

Oral carcinomas include those of the lip and oral cavity proper. The posterior margin of the oral cavity is the anterior faucial pillar on each side. The oral cavity has a rich lymphatic supply. Moreover lymphatic drainage is bilateral from a strip of midline tissue of the oral cavity and lip, which makes bilateral neck metastases more common in such tumours.

As well as primary tumours of the oral cavity, tumours of adjoining structures may present in the mouth. Examples are tumours of the maxillary sinus, salivary glands and oropharynx. Oral cancer is a relatively uncommon disease (the incidence being about two-thirds that of laryngeal cancer) occurring in older people. It is much more common in men and there is a pronounced geographical variation, these tumours being more common in India, Hong Kong and Singapore. The most important predisposing factors are tobacco smoke and alcohol, especially spirits. Lip cancer is more common in those exposed to large amounts of sunlight, and also in pipe smokers. The habit of betel nut chewing in India predisposes to buccal cancer. Carcinoma may arise in pre-existing leucoplakia or erythroplakia. Macroscopically these tumours appear ulcerative or exophytic (Fig. 22.1). There may be tethering of the tongue by infiltration of the tumour. The tongue and floor of the mouth are the most common sites of oral carcinoma. Microscopically more than 80% of tumours are squamous cell carcinoma. Tumours of the minor salivary glands and lymphoma are rarely encountered. Oral cancers have a habit of spreading into the tongue. An apparently small tumour of the tongue may in fact be widely infiltrating. Direct spread into the muscles of mastication can cause trismus. The periosteum of the mandible provides a quite effective barrier to tumour spread but in the edentulous mandible the tumour can

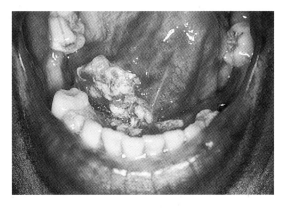

Fig. 22.1 Carcinoma of floor of mouth. Note the staining of the lips and poor dentition. The tongue must be moved out of the way to see the tumour.

spread more easily into bone from above. Lymphatic metastases occur in up to 40% of patients at presentation.

Oral cancer presents to the clinician with a persistent painful ulcer. If the alveolus is involved there may be a loose tooth, or patients may present to their general dental practitioner with ill-fitting dentures. Assessment involves an examination and biopsy, usually under general anaesthetic, and a panendoscopy to exclude a second primary tumour. Patients should have a chest X-ray, and orthopantomography (OPG) to assess mandibular invasion. CT or MRI may be indicated to assess the neck and help delineate the extent of tongue muscle invasion.

In principle, small tumours are treated by single modality therapy, while larger tumours are treated by combined radiotherapy and surgery. Most small lesions of the lip and oral cavity are managed by excision, with radiotherapy being kept in reserve for recurrent tumours. Larger tumours are treated by surgery to the primary tumour and neck (due to the high incidence of lymphatic metastases) and adjuvant postoperative radiotherapy. Surgical management of large oral cavity tumours presents a considerable challenge. Adequate access usually requires a mandibulotomy and the resulting surgical defect needs to be reconstructed with as little loss of function as possible. The use of microvascular free flaps for reconstruction has enhanced the options for restoration of function. It is important

Oral cavity

to avoid tethering of the tongue in order to retain normal speech and swallowing as far as possible.

The prognosis of oral cavity tumours depends upon the stage, the status of lymphatic metastases and the degree of differentiation between tumours. Lip cancer has a good prognosis, while the larger carcinomas of the floor of the mouth with lymphatic metastases carry a very poor one.

> **Key points**

> ➤ Periodontal disease is very common. Treatment is by aggressive topical therapy.
> ➤ Persistent oral ulcers should be biopsied to exclude malignancy.
> ➤ Leucoplakia represents a spectrum of disease but is abnormal and should be followed up and treated in order to reduce the development of malignant change.
> ➤ Small oral cancers can be treated by single modality therapy.
> ➤ The surgical treatment of large oral cancers presents a formidable surgical challenge and requires expertise in resection and appropriate reconstruction.

Salivary glands

23

Examination and general investigation of the salivary glands has been covered in Chapter 21. A careful history and examination will usually enable the clinician to move a long way towards diagnosis of diseases of the salivary glands and ducts. It is important to remember that there are several lymph nodes situated in and around the parotid gland, as well as in the submandibular triangle, and inflammatory or neoplastic disease can affect them.

INFLAMMATORY DISEASE

Parotitis

The mumps virus (which can also cause a hearing loss) is a common cause of a bilateral self-limiting parotitis in children. In adults it is most commonly seen in debilitated or immunocompromised patients, for example in diabetics. Such patients have poor oral hygiene and may be dehydrated. Xerostomia due to radiotherapy is a causative factor. It is caused by an ascending staphylococcal infection from the oral cavity and is usually unilateral. Chronic tuberculous infection (often by atypical forms) may develop in the surrounding lymph nodes. Infection of the gland may be secondary to obstruction of the duct by a calculus.

Clinically, patients complain of pain and swelling over the parotid gland. The pain and swelling are made worse by eating; spasm of the neighbouring muscles of mastication can cause trismus. Examination reveals a tender swelling of the entire gland and often an oedematous duct opening. Treatment is symptomatic. The patient is rehydrated if necessary, encouraged to consume citrus drinks to stimulate the flow of saliva and taught to massage the gland. A swab may be taken from the duct and an antistaphylococcal antibiotic prescribed. Surgical drainage of a parotid abscess is occasionally necessary.

In recurrent cases sialography may show sialectatic changes or a filling defect in the duct, suggesting a calculus, in which case surgical exploration of the duct is indicated.

Sialectasis and salivary stone disease

Sialectasis is a chronic condition of the major salivary glands in which the alveoli degenerate progressively and coalesce into cysts. Normal saliva production is disrupted and debris from the cysts passes along the ducts with saliva, blocking the ducts and leading to hypertrophy, stenosis and fibrosis. Stones form from a combination of stasis, obstruction and infection. Calculi are more of a clinical problem in the submandibular gland for the following reasons: Wharton's duct has a tortuous course, leading to a more sluggish flow of saliva, and the saliva in the submandibular gland is more mucinous, both of which encourage stone formation. These stones are invariably radio-opaque, unlike parotid calculi. It is most unlikely that stones form in a completely normal gland and there is usually evidence of sialectasis in glands that are removed for calculus.

Patients with sialectasis and stone disease present with recurrent swelling of the gland during and after eating. The submandibular gland is bound down by a tight fascia so any swelling causes considerable pain. If there are calculi, swelling may be followed by relief of symptoms and a foul taste in the mouth when a stone is expelled from the duct, releasing infected saliva. Alternatively a stone may fall back into the gland substance.

Examination may reveal a tender enlarged gland, and a stone may be palpable in the duct. A plain X-ray is always a useful investigation in submandibular disease, although parotid stones are usually radiolucent. If a stone is palpable well forward in Wharton's duct it can be excised under local anaesthetic; if the stone lies further back in the duct, the lingual nerve is at risk and intraoral removal should not be attempted.

If a patient continues to get recurrent symptoms after stone removal, or there are stones in the gland, the whole gland should be excised. Surgery on the parotid gland for inflammatory disease is a difficult procedure and should be avoided if at all possible.

SJÖGREN'S SYNDROME

Sjögren's syndrome is a connective tissue disease, associated with rheumatoid arthritis, which causes keratoconjunctivitis sicca (progressively dry, itchy eyes), xerostomia and often painful enlargement of one or both parotid glands. It is a disease of middle-aged women, and ocular and oral symptoms often dominate the clinical picture. The parotomegaly is usually intermittent to start with but becomes more established with time. This salivary enlargement is associated with lymphomatous transformation.

Diagnosis is clinical, supplemented by Schirmer's test, measurement of salivary flow rates and histological analysis of minor salivary gland tissue by a labial biopsy. There is periductal lymphocytic and plasmocytic infiltration and acinar destruction, often with associated non-specific sialadenitis.

Overall management is supervised by a rheumatologist. Careful attention is paid to oral and dental hygiene and salivary substitutes are prescribed. Surgery is indicated to alleviate the painful salivary gland enlargement or for diagnosis of lymphoma but is hazardous and should not be undertaken lightly.

TUMOURS

Major textbooks on salivary gland disease often contain long and complicated lists of tumours encountered in the salivary glands. A wide variety of pathology can be encountered but Box 23.1 provides a simplified classification of the more commonly encountered tumours that will be discussed in this chapter. Eighty per cent of tumours occur in the parotid gland, 80% of parotid tumours are benign and 80% of these benign tumours are pleomorphic adenomas. Malignant tumours are proportionately more common in the submandibular and minor salivary glands than in the parotid gland.

Benign

Pleomorphic adenomas (Fig. 23.1) present in young and middle-aged adults as a painless swelling in the parotid region, most commonly in the lower pole. Progressive enlargement takes place but the tumour is otherwise asymptomatic; benign tumours do not cause a facial palsy and are not painful. The tumour has a false capsule and wide excision with a cuff of normal tissue is thus necessary to prevent recurrence. If the lump is clinically in the superficial lobe without deep lobe extension, imaging is unnecessary, although fine needle aspiration cytology (FNAC) is helpful in diagnosis. Treatment is surgical via a superficial parotidectomy. The principles of this operation are first to expose the facial nerve as

---

■ Box 23.1

Simple classification of salivary gland tumours

Epithelial tumours
- Benign
  - Pleomorphic adenoma
  - Adenolymphoma (Warthin's tumour)
- Malignant
  - Mucoepidermoid carcinoma
  - Acinic cell carcinoma
  - Adenoid cystic carcinoma
  - Carcinoma in pleomorphic adenoma
  - Squamous cell carcinoma
  - Adenocarcinoma
  - Metastasis

Lymphoma

close to the stylomastoid foramen as possible, and then to follow it forward, dissecting off the tumour and surrounding normal tissue from the nerve until the tumour can be safely excised. This is much more likely to lead to preservation of facial nerve function than simple lumpectomy, which also has the serious disadvantage of seeding tumour, with disastrous consequences. The tumour can occasionally extend into the deep lobe (dumb-bell tumour), when a total parotidectomy preserving the facial nerve is indicated.

Adenolymphomas (Warthin's tumour) tend to occur in older people and are confined to the tail of the parotid; they may be variable in size and bilateral. Tendency to malignant change and recurrence is significantly less than with pleomorphic adenomas but treatment by superficial parotidectomy is the appropriate procedure in order to preserve the facial nerve.

Frey's syndrome (gustatory sweating) is a common complication of parotidectomy that may be troublesome to patients. Eating will precipitate pain and sweating (which may be profuse) in the parotid region, together with erythema. Frey's syndrome is probably caused by reinnervation of sympathetic branches by secretomotor fibres from the auriculotemporal nerve. Treatment may be unnecessary although application of anticholinergic cream can be successful. Surgical procedures include transmeatal tympanic neurectomy or denervating the skin by raising a large facial flap.

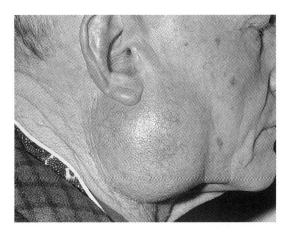

Fig. 23.1 Pleomorphic adenoma of the parotid gland.

Malignant

Malignant tumours are clinically distinguished from benign tumours by more rapid growth and pain. There may be an associated total or partial palsy but facial nerve function is often normal. Malignant change can occur in long-standing pleomorphic adenomas and this is characterised by pain or increased growth of an existing lump. The histological features are important in deciding management and determining prognosis. The mucoepidermoid and acinic cell tumours may fall into an intermediate or benign category, depending on the histological features. Adenoid cystic carcinoma has a tendency to perineural spread and skip lesions along the facial nerve.

FNAC may be very helpful in suspected malignant lesions and CT or MRI should be performed to help plan treatment, which is surgical. If facial nerve function is intact, the nerve should be preserved if possible. An en bloc neck dissection is indicated if there is metastatic lymphadenopathy, and facial skin may need to be sacrificed. Adjuvant postoperative radiotherapy may be helpful, although salivary gland tumours are not as radiosensitive as squamous cell carcinoma.

Follow-up of patients with malignant tumours needs to be lifelong; recurrence can occur many years after initial treatment.

Submandibular tumours

These are managed by sialadenectomy. If malignancy is suspected an extracapsular dissection is performed, with sacrifice of the mandibular branch of the facial nerve. Submandibular lymph nodes are excised in continuity and a neck dissection performed if lower node levels are involved.

Minor salivary gland tumours

These are usually malignant and carry a poor prognosis. They present as a hard non-ulcerating lesion in the oral cavity (Fig. 23.2) and are managed by wide excision, including resection of any potentially involved nerve as far proximally as possible. Reconstruction with local or distant flaps may be necessary to close any resulting defect.

Salivary glands

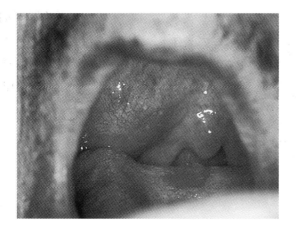

Fig. 23.2 Minor salivary gland tumour arising from the palate.

DROOLING

Excessive drooling is frequently encountered in cerebral palsy and other neurological disorders. It may cause problems with skin maceration around the mouth and chin as well as social isolation and a need for repeated changes of clothing or the wearing of bibs. It may also compromise the safety of using electrical communication aids.

Initially, advice on head posture, and therapy to improve jaw and lip closure as well as swallowing, may be beneficial. Anticholinergic drugs do reduce salivary flow but their complications make them inappropriate for indefinite use. Surgical redirection of salivary flow by submandibular duct transposition into the tonsillar fossae is effective in reducing drooling in over 80% of patients. Reported complications are minor and include sialadenitis, transient submandibular swelling and salivary retention cysts in the floor of the mouth. The incidence of such cysts may be reduced by sublingual gland excision at the same procedure. Parotid duct transposition has also been reported but carries the potential added complication of damage to branches of the facial and mandibular nerves. Alternatively, surgery to reduce salivary secretion may be undertaken. The complication of xerostomia with resulting dental caries may be a problem if salivary gland output is reduced to less than 5% of normal. Excision of the submandibular or parotid glands is associated with significant risk to branches of the lingual, hypoglossal and facial nerves and is rarely justified for drooling. Simple ligation of the parotid and submandibular ducts is frequently followed by painful prolonged swelling of the gland and cannot be advocated. Interruption of the parasympathetic nerve supply to the salivary glands will reduce secretion to a basal or resting level; via a tympanotomy, the chorda tympani, which supplies the submandibular and sublingual glands, and the tympanic plexus (Jacobson's nerve), which supplies the parotid gland, can conveniently both be divided at one procedure. However, because of the risk to hearing involved in middle ear surgery, procedures for the right and left ears should be staged and the operation is contraindicated in a patient with only one hearing ear. Reported success rates in reducing drooling vary between 50 and 90%.

> **► Key points**
> - ► Parotitis is a disease of debilitated patients and needs to be managed aggressively.
> - ► Sialectasis and stone disease is more common in the submandibular gland.
> - ► Calculi may be excised intraorally but only if anterior. Otherwise submandibular gland excision is necessary.
> - ► Most tumours are benign pleomorphic adenomas of the parotid.
> - ► Malignant tumours are characterised by rapid growth, pain and often facial palsy.
> - ► Treatment of salivary gland tumours is by facial nerve exposure and wide excision to avoid recurrence.

THE LARYNX, PHARYNX AND OESOPHAGUS

5

Anatomy and physiology of the larynx, pharynx and oesophagus

24

LARYNGEAL ANATOMY

Skeleton

The larynx consists of a cartilaginous framework bound together by ligaments and covered with muscle and mucous membrane. The cartilages of the larynx are usually referred to as paired and unpaired (Figs 24.1 and 24.2).

Unpaired cartilages

The epiglottis is a leaf-shaped cartilage which is attached to the base of the tongue by the glosso-epiglottic ligament and to the inner aspect of the thyroid cartilage. The thyroid cartilage is that which makes the prominence upon the front of the neck, known as the 'Adam's apple'. It consists of two wings, or alae, which are joined together in the midline anteriorly and extend backwards. In the front, at the junction of the alae, is the thyroid notch, which can be readily palpated. Posteriorly on the alae there are two processes, superior and inferior. Below the thyroid cartilage and articulating with the inferior processes is the cricoid cartilage. This is a closed circle of cartilage in the form of a signet ring, of which the signet or large portion is posterior. It is the only complete ring of cartilage in the respiratory tract. It is connected anteriorly with the thyroid cartilage by the cricothyroid membrane, which is also easily palpated. It is through this membrane that a cricothyroidotomy for the relief of airway obstruction is performed.

Paired cartilages

The most important of these are the arytenoid cartilages. They can rotate and slide on the cricoid and thus play an important part in the movement of the vocal cords. Each arytenoid has the shape of a three-sided pyramid.

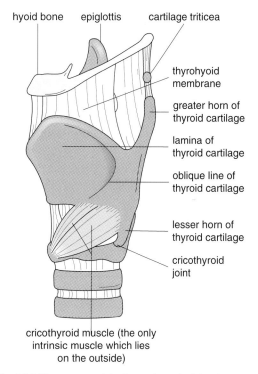

Fig. 24.1 The exterior of the larynx from the left side.

hyoid bone   epiglottis   cartilage triticea

thyrohyoid membrane

greater horn of thyroid cartilage

lamina of thyroid cartilage

oblique line of thyroid cartilage

lesser horn of thyroid cartilage

cricothyroid joint

cricothyroid muscle (the only intrinsic muscle which lies on the outside)

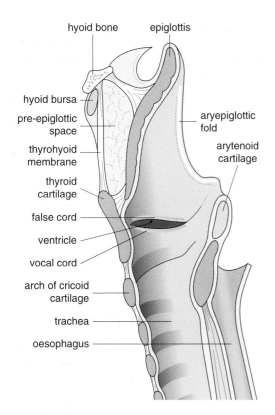

hyoid bone
epiglottis
hyoid bursa
pre-epiglottic space
thyrohyoid membrane
thyroid cartilage
false cord
ventricle
vocal cord
arch of cricoid cartilage
trachea
oesophagus
aryepiglottic fold
arytenoid cartilage

Fig. 24.2 Section of larynx.

The anterior process is known as the vocal process and the lateral as the muscular process. The vocal cords are attached to the vocal process anteriorly, while the muscular processes form the main attachment for those muscles activating the vocal cords in phonation and respiration. The aryepiglottic fold connects the arytenoid with the base of the epiglottis and forms the upper edge of the laryngeal inlet.

Interior of the larynx

Looking down upon the larynx, either with a mirror or endoscopically, the appearances are as illustrated in Figure 25.3. Examination of the larynx is described in Chapter 25.

The interior of the larynx is subdivided into the supraglottis, the glottis and the subglottis. The supraglottis and the subglottis have a much more abundant lymphatic drainage than the glottis,

which has implications for the management of cancer of these sites; the incidence of metastatic lymphadenopathy is higher in supraglottic and subglottic tumours, making the prognosis worse. The supraglottis is that part from the laryngeal inlet to the lower part of the laryngeal ventricle; the glottis comprises the vocal cords and the arytenoids; and the subglottis is that area below the cords. Between the epiglottis and the thyrohyoid membrane is the pre-epiglottic space. The false cords are rounded pink bands of mucosa lying above a space called the laryngeal ventricle. The lower lip of the ventricle is formed by a muscular bundle which is the true vocal cord. Seen from above, the cord looks narrow and white. Each cord looks like a band of white fibrous tissue stretching from front to back, but in reality all that is seen is the upper edge of a triangular bundle of muscular tissue (the conus elasticus), of which the outer edge is a thin condensation of fibrous tissue (Fig. 24.2).

The true cords are attached anteriorly in the midline to the posterior surface of the thyroid cartilage. Posteriorly they are attached to the vocal process of the arytenoid cartilages; the cords are in fact two-thirds membranous and one-third cartilaginous (Fig. 24.3).

Muscles

Two main muscle groups are often described in the larynx, the adductors and the abductors, although both groups act synergistically. The muscles are described according to their attachments (Fig. 24.3).

The cricothyroid muscle is the extrinsic muscle of the larynx and acts by extending the thyroid cartilage on the cricoid, thus tensing the vocal cord muscles. It is supplied by the external laryngeal nerve, unlike the intrinsic muscles which are supplied by the recurrent laryngeal nerve.

The thyroarytenoid muscle is the main internal tensor and lies alongside the vocal cord. Individual fibres insert into the vocal cord and are known as the vocalis muscle.

The lateral cricoarytenoid stretches from the lateral side of the cricoid cartilage to the muscular process of the arytenoid cartilage, and by contracting it rotates the arytenoid medially, bringing the cord towards the midline.

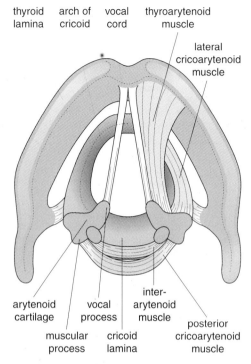

Fig. 24.3 Cartilages and intrinsic muscles of the larynx.

The posterior cricoarytenoid muscle is attached so that it rotates the arytenoid laterally, thus abducting the vocal cord. It is arguably the most important muscle in the body, being the only abductor of the cords and essential for normal respiration.

The interarytenoid muscle is attached to the bodies of the arytenoids; on contraction it adducts the vocal cords.

Nerve supply

The superior laryngeal nerve takes origin from the inferior ganglion of the vagus nerve and runs downwards to divide into the internal and external laryngeal nerves. The external nerve runs with the superior thyroid artery to supply the cricothyroid muscle. The internal laryngeal nerve pierces the thyrohyoid membrane and is sensory to the mucosa of the larynx above the level of the vocal cords.

The recurrent laryngeal nerve is a branch of the vagus nerve that has a differing course on each side for embryological reasons (it is the nerve of the sixth branchial arch). On the left side it passes under the aortic arch and ascends through the mediastinum in the tracheo-oesophageal groove to reach the neck, entering the larynx underneath the inferior constrictor muscle.

On the right side it does not descend into the thorax as far, looping round the subclavian artery, then passing back up into the neck. Because of its longer intrathoracic course, the left recurrent laryngeal nerve is more likely to be involved in cases of bronchogenic carcinoma. The recurrent laryngeal nerve is motor to all muscles of the larynx, apart from cricothyroid, and is sensory to the mucosa below the vocal cord.

LARYNGEAL FUNCTION

Table 24.1 lists the functions of the larynx.

PHARYNGEAL ANATOMY

The pharynx is divided into three areas: the nasopharynx, the oropharynx and the hypopharynx (or laryngopharynx). The boundaries of the nasopharynx are the basisphenoid above to a line at the level of the free border of the soft palate below; the oropharynx commences at the level of the soft palate and extends to the level of the tip of the epiglottis; the hypopharynx commences at the level of the tip of the epiglottis and extends to just below the level of the cricoid, where it is continuous with the oesophagus (Fig. 24.4).

The pharynx has several features common to all its parts. The mucous membrane throughout is stratified squamous epithelium. Inflammation of one part of the pharynx is readily transferred to the

Table 24.1 Functions of the larynx

Function	Produced by
Phonation	Vocal cords acting as vibrator
Protection of respiratory tract	Laryngeal elevation Epiglottis Sensory nerve supply (cough) Vocal cords

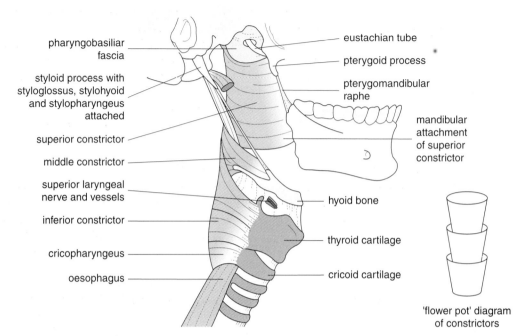

Fig. 24.4 Constrictors of the pharynx and associated structures. The three pharyngeal constrictors are related to each other so that they overlap like flower pots stacked up together.

others, so that all inflammatory conditions of the pharynx will potentially affect other areas of the pharynx (and often the larynx as well). The lymphoid tissue of the pharynx forms an important part of its structure and is involved in many diseases of the area.

Nasopharynx

The posterior wall of the nasopharynx arches forward into the roof, which is formed by the basisphenoid. At the junction of the roof and posterior wall is situated the aggregation of lymphoid tissue called the adenoids. Anteriorly the nasopharynx is in continuation with the posterior choanae of the nose; the posterior end of the septum and inferior turbinates are often visible on postnasal space examination. On the lateral wall there are the openings of the eustachian tubes: behind these are the eminences called the eustachian cushions and posterior to these are the fossae of Rosenmuller. These are deep fossae that extend laterally below the skull base; they are in close proximity to the lower cranial nerves. Nasopharyngeal carcinoma commonly arises from the fossa of Rosenmuller so

may present late with cranial nerve palsies if it extends laterally.

Oropharynx

The nasopharynx and oropharynx are separated by the strong, mobile, membranous-muscular soft palate, posterior to which is the nasopharyngeal isthmus. The uvula hangs from the soft palate and is occasionally bifid. A submucous cleft may extend forward in such patients. The palate may look normal but the abnormal cleft is felt on palpation. Two folds of muscle and mucosa stretch down on each side from the palate to meet the lateral border of the tongue. These are the pillars of the fauces; between them lie the palatine tonsils. The anterior faucial pillars form the junction between oropharynx and oral cavity. Embedded into the tongue base are the lingual tonsils. The adenoids, palatine and lingual tonsils form Waldeyer's ring, a circle of lymphoid tissue surrounding the opening to the digestive tract. This area has a role in the priming of lymphocytes for antigens during the early years of life. There are many aggregations of lymphoid tissue on the posterior wall of the oropharynx which can be seen when inflamed.

The dorsum of the tongue can be followed down until it reaches the base of the epiglottis. Between the base of the tongue and the front of the epiglottis lie two spaces known as the valleculae. They are divided in the midline by the glossoepiglottic ligament and posterolaterally by the pharyngoepiglottic ligaments.

Hypopharynx

This is the part of the pharynx that lies behind the larynx. The pyriform fossae commence behind the pharyngoepiglottic ligaments. These fossae are triangular-shaped potential spaces with their apices inferiorly formed by the bulk of the larynx projecting posteriorly. Their old name of 'lateral food channel' is a particularly good descriptive term of their site and function.

Posterior to the larynx is the postcricoid area, site of the only head and neck squamous tumours that are more common in women. The posterior pharyngeal wall completes the hypopharynx, and the oesophagus commences at the cricopharyngeus, which lies 15 cm from the upper incisor teeth.

Muscles

The pharynx can be regarded as a muscular funnel suspended from the skull base and supported by attachments to the mandible and the laryngeal skeleton. The most powerful muscles are the superior, middle and inferior constrictors, which, contracting in succession, squeeze food downwards to the oesophageal entrance. The lower fibres of the inferior constrictor muscle are called the cricopharyngeus and completely encircle the pharynx. This muscle remains tonically contracted except when it relaxes as part of the swallowing reflex, thus acting as the upper oesophageal sphincter. Posteriorly, between the cricopharyngeus and the other fibres of the inferior constrictor, lies a thin membrane where there is an absence of muscle support. This is called Killian's dehiscence and it is of importance in the development of pharyngeal pouches.

Because the pharynx must allow air to flow between nose and larynx, and food from mouth to oesophagus, a complex system of muscle coordination is required to close the nasopharyngeal isthmus and

the laryngeal inlet at appropriate times, and so keep these two functions separated.

The muscles providing vertical movement are chiefly the stylopharyngeus and the palatopharyngeus. Those which control the soft palate are the levator palati, the tensor palati and the palatoglossus. Salpingopharyngeus, as well as tensor palati and levator palati, controls the patency of the eustachian tube.

Nerve supply

The sensory nerve supply of the nasopharynx is from branches of the maxillary nerve. A pharyngeal plexus lies on the lateral wall of the constrictors, deriving fibres from the glossopharyngeal and vagus nerves and the cervical sympathetic trunk. From here sensory nerves from the glossopharyngeal nerve supply the oropharynx. Branches of the internal laryngeal nerve supply the hypopharynx. The motor supply to the constrictors is from the vagus, but the cricopharyngeus is supplied directly by the recurrent laryngeal nerve.

Waldeyer's ring

See p. 177.

OESOPHAGEAL ANATOMY

The oesophagus is a muscular tube connecting the pharynx to the stomach. It commences at the cricopharyngeus (the upper oesophageal sphincter) and enters the stomach at the gastro-oesophageal junction (the lower oesophageal sphincter). It is 25 cm in length and has a short cervical segment, a larger intrathoracic section and a small intra-abdominal part. The oesophagus is lined by stratified squamous epithelium, with an abrupt change to columnar epithelium at the gastro-oesophageal junction. It has an outer longitudinal muscle coat and an inner circular coat that is striated in the upper third, mixed in the middle third and smooth muscle in the lower third. The striated muscle is supplied by the recurrent laryngeal nerve and the rest by the parasympathetic system.

The upper oesophageal sphincter at the level of the cricopharyngeus remains tonically closed except when swallowing (see below). The lower sphincter is more of a 'physiological' sphincter that relies on a variety of mechanisms to maintain the pressure above that of the stomach. These include a 'pinch-cock' effect of the muscles of the diaphragm, the thoracoabdominal pressure gradient and the angle of the oesophagogastric junction.

The oesophagus is the narrowest part of the alimentary tract and has three recognisable constrictions, which is of clinical importance when managing patients with obstructing foreign bodies (see Box 24.1). It is also important to know that the oesophagus curves anteriorly in its intrathoracic course and deviates to the left as it goes through the diaphragm into the stomach.

SWALLOWING

Swallowing is a complicated integrated process whereby a bolus is transferred from the buccal cavity to the stomach. A variety of different muscles and many nerves, somatic and visceral, afferent and efferent, are involved. At the same time, it is necessary to protect the airway and prevent food passing into the respiratory tract.

Swallowing can be divided into three phases:

1. oral
2. pharyngeal
3. oesophageal.

The oral phase can be further divided into two components, the preparatory and the propulsive phases. The preparatory phase involves lip closure, jaw movement, buccal tone, tongue movement and prevention of premature spillage of food into the oropharynx. Food is broken down into an appropriate consistency and is mixed with saliva, which lubricates the bolus and starts the digestive process.

Good coordination and tongue mobility are essential to this phase. Once an adequate bolus has been created, the palatoglossal sphincter opens and the tongue pumps the bolus into the oropharynx by sequential contraction along the palate.

The pharyngeal phase is complex and important because of the interaction with the larynx. Four neuromuscular activities are associated with this phase:

1. velopharyngeal closure to prevent reflux into the nasopharynx
2. pharyngeal peristalsis
3. airway protection
4. cricopharyngeal opening.

Gravity and lingual propulsion play a more important role than pharyngeal peristalsis in bolus transit through the pharynx. Peristalsis clears the residue left following the gravitational transit. Laryngeal elevation opens the pharyngeal inlet, helping to suck food down into the pharynx; it also plays a role in opening the upper oesophageal sphincter (as well as cricopharyngeal relaxation) by drawing the cricoid anteriorly. Airway protection involves laryngeal elevation and three sphincters – the epiglottis, the aryepiglottic fold and the true vocal cords – of which the last is most important. The epiglottis closes like a trap door and diverts the bulk of the food bolus around the larynx into the lateral food channels (pyriform fossae). During this time (which is only a fraction of a second) respiration ceases.

The oesophageal phase starts as the bolus passes through the upper oesophageal sphincter and ends as it enters the stomach. The bolus passes partly by gravity and partly with the help of oesophageal peristalsis. This phase takes about 10 seconds.

■ **Box 24.1**

Constrictions in the oesophagus

- At 15 cm from upper incisor teeth: cricopharyngeus
- At 23 cm from upper incisor teeth: oesophagus crossed by left main bronchus
- At 40 cm from upper incisor teeth: pierces diaphragm (lower sphincter)

► **Key points**

► The larynx and pharynx are intimately related anatomically and physiologically.
► The larynx has a dual role: voice production and as a sphincter to protect the airway.
► The pharynx is a complex area of muscles supplied by several nerves which act synergistically to control the process of swallowing.

Examination and assessment of the larynx and pharynx

INDIRECT LARYNGOSCOPY

Indirect laryngoscopy (Fig. 25.1) is a simple procedure, within the capabilities of any well-trained practitioner prepared to give some time to its practice. Gentleness on the part of the examiner and relaxation on the part of the patient are important for success, as is giving the patient a full explanation of the procedure beforehand.

Good illumination is absolutely essential: a head mirror or head light can be used for this purpose. The patient should sit upright with the head forward, while the examiner sits in front of the patient or on the patient's left side (assuming the examiner is right-handed). If the patient has an active gag reflex, use of an anaesthetic spray is helpful.

The patient is asked to protrude the tongue, any dentures having been removed, and it is grasped with a gauze swab. The thumb may be above or below the tongue according to the preference of the examiner, but one finger should be able to raise the upper lip if necessary. The grip should be firm but gentle, and the tongue should on no account be pinched but rather rolled over the finger below it. Care must be taken to protect the frenulum from damage by lower teeth.

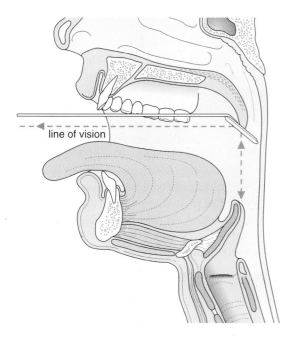

Fig. 25.1a Indirect laryngoscopy showing direction of light beam upon the larynx.

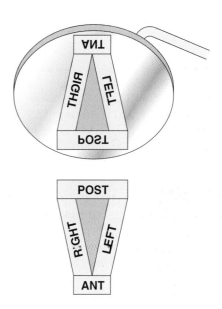

Fig. 25.1b Demonstration of how the image is reversed in the laryngeal mirror in indirect laryngoscopy.

A large size of laryngeal mirror is warmed and placed firmly but gently on the soft palate just above the base of the uvula. The light is then directed to the various parts of the larynx and hypopharynx by tilting the mirror, but the mirror should not actually be moved from its place on the soft palate or the patient may gag. The patient is asked to breathe easily and steadily throughout. It is better for the patient if several short examinations are made than if the clinician tries to see everything in one attempt.

The first structure to come into view is the epiglottis, which usually overhangs the interior of the larynx. The epiglottis sometimes overhangs to such a degree that it is impossible to view the larynx with a mirror, and flexible nasolaryngoscopy is used. The valleculae and tongue base are then viewed, followed by the aryepiglottic folds and pyriform fossae. Each structure is examined in turn and note is made of any redness of the mucous membrane, swelling, oedema, excess of secretions, ulceration or any other abnormality.

To examine the interior of the larynx it helps if the patient tries to say 'ee'. The epiglottis will rise and the larynx comes into view.

Interior of the larynx

Having exposed the larynx, it is possible to study the structures within it (Fig. 25.2). The aryepiglottic

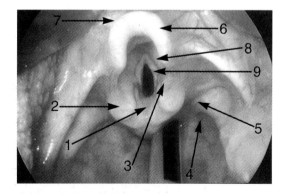

Fig. 25.2 View of a child's larynx from above.
(1) Interarytenoid region; (2) arytenoid cartilage;
(3) aryepiglottic fold; (4) pyriform fossa; (5) pharyngoepiglottic fold; (6) epiglottis; (7) vallecula; (8) false cords; (9) true cords.

folds are looked at first, and then the arytenoids themselves. These should be smooth and symmetrical, and a healthy pink. The false cords are examined next: they should appear equal, and should not overhang or conceal the true cords below. If they do, they should be regarded as abnormal. Their surface should be smooth. The true cords should be white, smooth and glistening, with a slight degree of moisture, but there should be no appearance of secretion lying on them. It is important to note any asymmetry, including irregularity of the edges, nodule formation or ulceration. In some cases glistening irregularities are seen, and these are probably lumps of mucus. The anterior ends of the vocal cords (the anterior commisure) are sometimes difficult to see. A certain amount of redundant mucosa may be regarded as normal in the interarytenoid region. In many instances the upper part of the trachea may be visible.

Movement of the vocal cords

The final part of indirect laryngoscopy is inspection of the movement of the larynx and vocal cords. It is important to ascertain if the vocal cords are moving normally or if there is any fixation or paralysis. It must be remembered that the image is a mirror image and therefore reversed. The first abnormality that may appear to the inexperienced examiner may be an inequality in the excursion of the cords; this, however, is more apparent than real because of the tilting of the mirror, which gives a distorted view. The mirror must therefore be held so that the image is centralised and vertical as far as possible.

The first position examined (Fig. 25.3) is that of quiet respiration. In this the cords should lie moderately separated, and equidistant from the midline. On inspiration they move outwards a small distance, and on expiration they move in again, but do not reach the midline. On forced inspiration the outward excursion is much greater. Phonation brings the cords together, though a slight chink can still be seen, and the cords vibrate rapidly or more slowly, according to the note produced. In the act of coughing the cords come closely into apposition before the air is expelled.

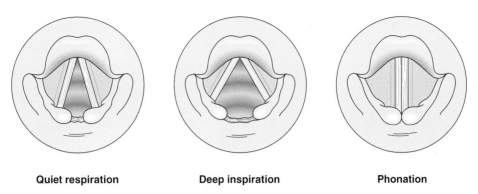

Quiet respiration   Deep inspiration   Phonation

Fig. 25.3 Appearances of the vocal cords on mirror laryngoscopy: quiet respiration; deep inspiration; phonation.

Quality of the voice

In some patients the voice is of poor volume, breathy but not rough. Owing to excessive air wastage much energy goes into the production of comparatively little sound. Such patients may be found to have a paralysis.

In other patients the voice is truly rough in quality and this roughness often corresponds to the degree of irregularity of the vocal cord on which the lesion is situated. It is in these instances that the voice may properly be described as 'hoarse'.

PHARYNGEAL EXAMINATION

The hypopharynx is examined with the larynx during indirect laryngoscopy. The oropharynx is best studied by depressing the tongue with a rigid tongue depressor. An angled postnasal space mirror can then be gently introduced to view the nasopharynx.

FIBREOPTIC EXAMINATION

The flexible fibreoptic laryngoscope (Fig. 25.4) is now commonly used in the assessment of laryngeal and pharyngeal disease. A good mirror examination provides a better view than fibreoptic examination but the latter is especially useful in those with an overhanging epiglottis and a prominent gag reflex. It can be used in young infants and has the added advantage of providing a comprehensive view of at least one nasal cavity and the postnasal space as well as the larynx and pharynx. A video recording can

be made for feedback to patients and a teaching arm or monitor is useful for teaching purposes. For a description of the technique of flexible nasendoscopy, see Chapter 17.

VIDEOSTROBOSCOPY

A wide-bore rigid 90° fibreoptic endoscope can be passed transorally to view the larynx. Videostroboscopy can be used in conjunction with this instrument to assess vocal cord function in fine detail. By adjusting the speed of the flash, the movement of the vocal cords can be slowed, or even 'frozen', giving a detailed picture of the cycle of vocal cord movement. This is especially useful in patients undergoing speech therapy and is also finding an important role in assessing the depth of invasion of early laryngeal carcinoma.

Finally, the neck should be examined in all patients in whom an indirect laryngoscopy or nasendoscopy is undertaken.

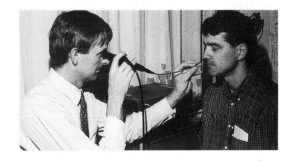

Fig. 25.4 Fibreoptic laryngoscopy.

ASSESSMENT OF PHARYNGEAL FUNCTION

Some aspects of pharyngeal function can be assessed directly by asking the patient to swallow milk or a coloured liquid while the examiner observes the hypopharynx with a fibreoptic nasolaryngoscope. Swallowing can be more completely evaluated using the radiographic technique of videofluoroscopy (cine swallow). Unlike a normal barium swallow, when the patient swallows the contrast material the entire process is continuously recorded on video-tape. When replayed in slow motion the flow of contrast can be assessed.

> **Key points**
>
> ➤ With practice, indirect laryngoscopy is an easily learned and valuable technique.
> ➤ Gentleness by the examiner and confidence from the patient are the key to successful examination.
> ➤ Asymmetric findings on indirect laryngoscopy are always abnormal.
> ➤ Fibreoptic nasolaryngoscopy is complementary to mirror examination.

Tonsils and adenoids

26

WALDEYER'S RING

Waldeyer's ring is a ring of lymphoid tissue at the entrance to the aerodigestive tract. It consists of the adenoids, the pharyngeal tonsils ('the tonsils') and the lingual tonsils, which are embedded in the posterior third of the tongue. The size of the tonsils and adenoids varies with age: physiological hypertrophy is maximal between the ages of 2 and 5 years; involution, especially of the adenoids, is advanced by puberty.

The adenoid tissue is disposed in bilateral vertical ridges on the posterosuperior wall of the nasopharynx, laterally abutting the eustachian cushions (Fig. 26.1). The adenoids have no capsule. The tonsils are situated on either side of the oropharynx, the medial surface of each is exposed in the pharynx and pitted by a number of crypts lined with epithelium. A supratonsillar fossa lies above each tonsil, a developmental remnant of the second pharyngeal pouch. On all but its superficial aspect the tonsil is surrounded by a dense pseudocapsule of fibrous tissue and then by loose areolar tissue, separating it from the pharyngobasilar fascia covering the muscles of the tonsil bed. This capsule facilitates tonsillectomy.

Waldeyer's ring forms an initial site of contact with incoming organisms. The crypts and folds of the tonsils and adenoids collect antigens for immune processing. Sensitised B lymphocytes produce IgA locally and at other sites; T lymphocytes form part of the immune system acting against certain viruses. However, the tonsils and adenoids may themselves become the focus of troublesome infections and their removal does not appear to compromise immune function.

ADENOIDS

Adenoids that are large in relation to the nasopharynx may cause nasal obstruction, hyponasal speech, snoring and mouth breathing with excessive nasal discharge, often purulent. The child may be described as 'always having a cold'. The enlargement may be physiological hypertrophy or a result of chronic adenoiditis. If other conditions that cause nasal obstruction and rhinorrhoea (such as atopic rhinitis) have been excluded, adenoidectomy

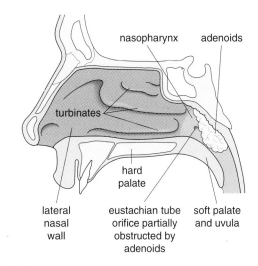

Fig. 26.1 Adenoids.

Tonsils and adenoids

may be helpful in the management of these symptoms. Not all mouth breathing is caused by adenoids however; many children with patent nasal airways habitually mouth breathe and this habit will not be altered by adenoidectomy.

The relationship between adenoidal hypertrophy or infection and middle ear problems remains controversial. There is, however, evidence that adenoidectomy in children hastens the resolution of otitis media with effusion and reduces the frequency of acute otitis media. These clinical findings therefore constitute accepted indications for adenoidectomy.

The diagnosis of adenoidal hypertrophy is mainly based on the history and an assessment of nasal patency. The appearance on posterior rhinoscopy using a nasopharyngeal mirror may be contributory but this examination is often difficult in children. Adenoid size can also be assessed with the flexible nasendoscope. A lateral soft tissue radiograph of the nasopharynx may be misleading as the apparent size of the airway can vary with the phase of respiration.

Adenoidal enlargement is rare after puberty: the differential diagnosis of a mass in the nasopharynx includes angiofibroma and nasopharyngeal carcinoma; any tissue removed in older children or adults should be examined histologically.

Adenoidectomy

This is carried out under general anaesthesia with an orotracheal tube in position; a pack may be placed around the tube to protect the airway. The mouth is held open using a gag. The adenoid pad should then be examined digitally or with a mirror. Adenoidectomy using a curette to shave the tissue off the nasopharyngeal wall has been the traditional technique; a postnasal pack is then inserted for a few minutes to control the bleeding. Postoperative haemorrhage occurs rarely but necessitates a return to the operating theatre for another postnasal pack to be placed; this is left in position for 24–48 hours. A suction diathermy technique minimises the risk of haemorrhage; this is significant with the trend towards day case surgery.

There is a risk of hypernasality after adenoidectomy if it is carried out after cleft palate repair or in the presence of a submucous cleft palate. The latter is suspected if the uvula is bifid and there is notching of the hard palate.

TONSILS

On inspection the appearance of the tonsils is variable and does not correlate well with symptoms of recurrent tonsillitis. Examination between attacks of tonsillitis is therefore of limited value in making a decision about tonsillectomy. The tonsils may be deeply recessed behind the anterior pillar of the fauces and almost invisible, or stand out prominently as if on a broad-based pedicle. Both are normal; the variation is simply one of anatomy. To a great extent it is the history rather than the appearance which is important in the management of tonsillitis.

Acute tonsillitis

This is a generalised inflammation of the tonsils, usually accompanied by a degree of inflammation of the fauces and pharynx. The infecting agent may be bacterial or viral. Rhinoviruses, adenoviruses and enteroviruses are probably responsible for about 50% of acute tonsillitis. Bacterial infection may be caused by Streptococci, Pneumococci, Staphylococci and *Haemophilus influenzae.* A throat swab may not determine the primary causative organism because of colonisation of the pharynx with commensals.

The most common symptom is a very sore throat. There may be a desire to swallow because of excessive secretions – swallowing tends to exacerbate the pain and patients tend to be anorexic. Fever and malaise are common and a young child can be quite ill. Referred otalgia and mesenteric adenitis producing abdominal pain are not unusual.

The tonsils are swollen and the overlying mucous membrane bright red. The uvula and soft palate may be oedematous. The crypts become filled with debris, desquamated epithelium and pus. The pus exudes on to the surface of the tonsil, producing the characteristic appearance of follicular tonsillitis. In very severe infection a patchy, fibrinous 'membrane' may appear over the surface of the tonsils – 'membranous tonsillitis'. The cervical glands are frequently enlarged and tender. Resolution of the infection usually takes place over 1–2 weeks and the tonsils revert to their previous condition; resolution may, however, be incomplete and residual infection persist.

Complications

Peritonsillar abscess or quinsy is the most common complication of acute tonsillitis; retropharyngeal abscess may also occur. Infection with the beta-haemolytic Streptococcus may result in the sequelae of scarlet fever, rheumatic fever or glomerulo-nephritis. Serological testing for infectious mononucleosis should be considered in patients where ulceration and glandular enlargement are marked features, especially in the older child or when symptoms persist.

Treatment

An adequate intake of fluids should be encouraged. Symptomatic treatment, including appropriate systemic analgesia, anaesthetic throat lozenges and antiseptic gargles, may be beneficial. Antibiotic treatment is indicated if symptoms are severe, penicillin or erythromycin being the first line of treatment but, if there is no response, beta-lactamase-producing organisms or anaerobes may be implicated and a broader spectrum antibiotic necessary.

Chronic tonsillitis

Chronic tonsillitis may be caused by repeated attacks of acute tonsillitis in which permanent damage has been done to the tonsil; it can also occur when resolution has been incomplete. Organisms may lie dormant for a short or a long time and produce acute symptoms again when a patient's general resistance is lowered for some reason. The tonsils in these patients are often deceptively innocent-looking and are sometimes so fibrosed down that they are difficult to see. Glandular fever not infrequently produces this type of permanent damage.

Peritonsillar abscess (quinsy)

A peritonsillar abscess generally arises as a complication of acute tonsillitis. Infection passes through the tonsil capsule into the loose peritonsillar layer of areolar tissue, where it causes cellulitis and then an abscess. Severe sore throat develops, associated with acute dysphagia and drooling. Otalgia on the affected side is common. There is generalised malaise and dehydration. Trismus is always a feature and this may make detailed inspection of the pharynx difficult. The soft palate bulges downwards and forwards and the uvula is displaced from the midline. The mucous membrane is red and oedematous, but the tonsils themselves may appear normal. The jugulodigastric lymph node in the neck may be enlarged and tender.

During the stage of cellulitis, prior to abscess formation, antibiotics may be effective. If not, incision and drainage will be necessary, and this is performed in the clinic. A guarded knife is fashioned by winding tape around the blade about a centimetre from its point as a precaution against entering too deeply. It is introduced into the abscess through the most prominent part of the soft palate, and the opening is then widened using sinus forceps. Where no obvious point of fluctuation can be found, a vertical line is taken from the point at which the anterior pillar joins the tongue and a horizontal line through the base of the uvula; the incision is made at the intersection of these two lines (Fig. 26.2). Relief of symptoms is instantaneous but should be followed by a complete course of appropriate antibiotics.

Prior local anaesthetic spray or injection is not effective in preventing the pain of incision and drainage, probably because of the inflammation. It also carries a small risk of subsequent unconscious inhalation of pus. General anaesthesia may be complicated by rupture of the abscess by the anaesthetic tube and, while not absolutely contraindicated, should be undertaken with caution. A 'quinsy' tonsillectomy is rarely necessary but may relieve airway obstruction complicating bilateral quinsies.

Tonsillectomy

Box 26.1 lists the indications for tonsillectomy.

The patient should be generally well and have been free of throat symptoms for at least 2 weeks. Any tendency to abnormal bleeding should have been investigated and its significance established.

The procedure is performed under general

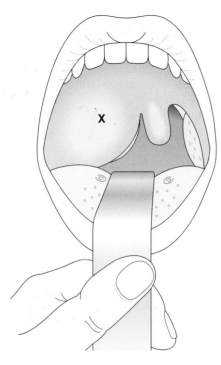

Fig. 26.2 Draining a quinsy. The quinsy is entered with forceps or a guarded knife at point X and opened. It must be emphasised that in reality there is severe trismus and the view is limited. Furthermore, if there is no trismus there is no quinsy. The swelling in these circumstances may be a tumour and should not be incised.

■ Box 26.1

Indications for tonsillectomy

- Recurrent tonsillitis – if this is well documented, frequent and sufficiently severe as to interfere with the patient's normal activities
- Peritonsillar abscess – if it follows a history of recurrent tonsillitis or occurs on more than one occasion
- Obstructive sleep apnoea syndrome
- Unilateral enlarged tonsil in an adult or ulceration of the tonsil – for histological assessment
- Less definite indications for tonsillectomy are acute rheumatic fever and acute nephritis; tonsillectomy may be beneficial in reducing the risk of further attacks if streptococcal tonsillitis has been the cause

anaesthesia with endotracheal intubation or a laryngeal mask to protect the airway. The patient is supine, the neck extended and the surgeon sits at the head wearing a head light. Dissection tonsillectomy is probably the procedure of choice, although guillotine tonsillectomy is still performed in some centres. The former can be undertaken using a traditional combination of sharp and blunt dissection or using monopolar or bipolar diathermy or the KTP laser. The mucosa is incised and the tonsil capsule identified. The tonsil is separated from its bed, dissecting through the loose areolar tissue external to the tonsil capsule (Fig. 26.3). A snare or a tie may be used at the lower pole of the palatine tonsil to separate it from the lingual tonsil. Bleeding is controlled by ligatures or bipolar diathermy. At the end of the procedure any blood clot in the nasopharynx should be aspirated through the nose, as it may oth-

erwise be aspirated into the trachea on recovery from anaesthesia.

Postoperatively, the patient's condition, including pulse and blood pressure, are regularly monitored. The surgeon should be alert to the possibility of bleeding: repeated swallowing may be a sign of this. Regular analgesia is administered (avoiding aspirin) and swallowing encouraged. A normal diet should be resumed as soon as possible. Usually patients are fit for discharge from hospital on the first postoperative day. They should be warned about referred otalgia and the risk of secondary haemorrhage.

Complications

Primary or reactionary haemorrhage This occurs within 24 hours of surgery and may be catastrophic. It is caused by inadequate or incomplete haemostasis at the time of surgery, by subsequent vasodilatation and reopening of the vessels, or by the slipping of ligatures.

If haemorrhage occurs, the patient must first be resuscitated; blood samples should be taken for crossmatching of blood and to rule out any clotting abnormality. The throat is then examined; if there is a clot on the tonsil bed, this may be keeping an underlying vessel open and perpetuating bleeding,

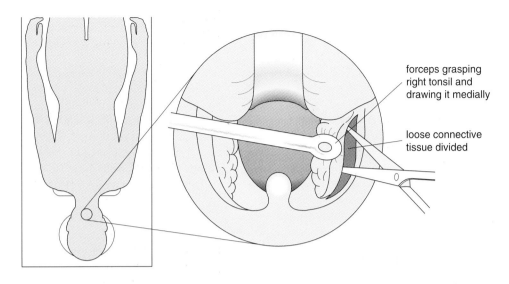

forceps grasping
right tonsil and
drawing it medially

loose connective
tissue divided

Fig. 26.3 Technique of tonsillectomy. The patient is supine on the table with a sandbag under the shoulders and a head ring under the head. The surgeon sits at the head of the table. A very shallow incision is made in the mucosa to expose the tonsil capsule. The tonsil is then firmly grasped and blunt dissection proceeds in the loose layer of connective tissue between tonsil and pharyngeal wall. A snare finally separates the lower pole of the tonsil from the lingual tonsil.

so it should be removed using a gloved finger. One in 1000 adrenaline solution on a cotton-wool ball is then applied topically to the tonsil bed and may be effective in preventing further haemorrhage. If not, the blood vessel responsible must be ligated and this will necessitate a return to the operating theatre.

Secondary haemorrhage This may occur between 5 and 10 days after tonsillectomy and is caused by separation of the slough which has formed on the tonsil bed. It is more likely if the slough has built up in a patient who has not been swallowing adequately. The volume of blood loss is usually small.

Despite the minor nature of this complication in most patients, it must be managed cautiously as there is the potential for a serious haemorrhage. Resuscitation is not usually necessary but the patient should be admitted to hospital overnight and blood cross-matched. Local treatment by removal of the clot and application of topical adrenaline is successful in most cases. Oral antibiotics should be administered and seem to be effective in preventing recurrence. Only rarely does a secondary haemorrhage necessitate a return to the operating theatre but, when it does, infection and granulations

make simple ligation of the bleeding vessel difficult and it may be necessary to suture the pillars together over a piece of commercially produced haemostatic agent to achieve haemostasis.

OBSTRUCTIVE SLEEP APNOEA SYNDROME

Obstructive sleep apnoea syndrome (OSAS) is increasingly recognised in childhood; it occurs most frequently between the ages of 2 and 5 years. Presenting features include stertor, loud snoring, irregular respiration, increased respiration, apnoeas, arousals, enuresis, daytime hypersomnolence, behavioural disorders and growth retardation. In severe cases alveolar hypoventilation results in hypoxia and hypercapnia, following which pulmonary hypertension, cor pulmonale, cardiac dysrhythmias, acute cardiorespiratory failure and sudden death may ensue.

Physiological hypertrophy of the tonsils and adenoids is the most common cause of OSAS in children. In conditions in which the nasopharynx is small, such as Apert's syndrome, Crouzon's syndrome and Down's syndrome, the risk of airway compromise is increased. A large tongue – as occurs in Pierre

Robin sequence and the mucopolysaccharidoses – or a small mandible may also precipitate OSAS. Investigation is directed towards establishing the cause, severity and any medical complications that may have occurred. The use of a validated questionnaire may be helpful. Lateral neck radiography, lateral cephalometry, CT and MRI of the airway may be indicated. Polysomnography will detect sleep apnoea syndrome and distinguish between obstructive and central types. Overnight pulse oximetry alone should be used with caution as the absence of significant desaturation does not exclude dangerously increased upper airway resistive loads during sleep. Chest radiography and electrocardiography will show signs consistent with pulmonary hypertension and cor pulmonale, if these are present.

In an otherwise well child with classical symptoms of OSAS, adenotonsillectomy is the first step in management; this will often relieve the obstruction, even if a small nasopharynx or other anatomical variant is the predisposing factor and adenotonsillar hypertrophy is not the primary cause of the problem. If adenotonsillectomy fails to control symptoms, further investigations should be undertaken. Other options for treatment include maxillary or mandibular advancement, continuous positive airways pressure via a face mask or nasal prong, and tracheostomy.

In children, polysomnography is difficult, inconvenient and expensive, requiring specialised equipment and personnel. Although it is the 'gold standard' investigation for OSAS, it is usually reserved for equivocal cases where complicating central apnoea is suspected or there are contraindications to adenotonsillectomy. It can also be used after interventions to monitor the success of treatment.

> ► **Key points**
>
> ► Adenoids are not always the cause of nasal obstruction and rhinorrhoea in children.
> ► Consider diagnosis of glandular fever in teenagers and young adults with 'membranous tonsillitis'.
> ► Although uncommon, serious complications of tonsillectomy may occur.
> ► Obstructive sleep apnoea syndrome in children is an important diagnosis not to miss.

Infections of the pharynx and larynx

27

PHARYNGITIS

While non-specific pharyngitis is very common, other infections of the pharynx are extremely rare. Indeed, some diseases described in this chapter – such as diphtheria – are almost unknown in the developed world but are still encountered in developing countries. The acute diseases most commonly involve the oropharynx, so are readily seen on examination.

The role of nasal disease, and less commonly gastro-oesophageal reflux, must be remembered in the pathogenesis of pharyngeal disorders. Postnasal drip, especially when infected, can cause acute and chronic inflammation of the larynx and pharynx and this link emphasises the importance of performing a full otorhinolaryngological examination on all patients presenting to an outpatient clinic.

Acute

This may be a simple acute pharyngitis or caused by an infective agent. It may be caused by cold air, irritation from fumes at work, a smoky atmosphere or postnasal drip, or be secondary to gastro-oesophageal reflux. Infective pharyngitis is generally streptococcal and may occur in outbreaks in schools or workplaces.

In simple acute pharyngitis the patient complains of an irritation and rawness of the throat with slight pain on swallowing. This may become chronic and persistent but generally resolves once the cause is removed, helped by simple measures such as steam inhalations and paracetamol gargles.

In infective pharyngitis the patient is more ill, with severe odynophagia and lymphadenopathy. On examination the posterior fauces, soft palate and posterior pharyngeal wall are red and inflamed; the aggregates of lymphoid tissue on the posterior pharyngeal wall stand out as brighter patches of inflammation, and mucopus may be seen on the mucous membranes. Treatment is symptomatic in mild cases, as described above. Patients should be strongly encouraged to stop smoking if they are smokers. If severe, and there is systemic upset, an antibiotic such as amoxycillin should be prescribed.

Chronic

This is a more chronic low grade problem than acute pharyngitis. It is generally due to irritation of the mucous membrane by an endogenous irritant such as postnasal drip or gastro-oesophageal reflux, or exogenous irritants such as smoke or fumes in the workplace. Chronic dental sepsis may also be a cause. The symptoms are generally those of a sore throat and an irritation like that of a foreign body. The mucous membrane may be red and congested with prominent lymphoid follicles.

Treatment is aimed at resolving the endogenous cause and eliminating irritants in the atmosphere, in particular stopping the patient from smoking. Symptomatic treatment with paracetamol gargles and steam inhalations as well as reassurance usually suffices.

Infectious mononucleosis (glandular fever)

This is a generalised disorder which causes a pharyngotonsillitis. It is caused by the Epstein–Barr virus, which is spread by droplet transmission. Patients usually have a prodromal illness followed by severe sore throat associated with odynophagia, malaise and massive bilateral lymphadenopathy. On examination the tonsils are covered by a characteristic plaque. There may be associated petechial haemorrhages as well as hepatoslenomegaly, encephalitis and cranial nerve palsies.

Diagnosis is based on the presence of atypical T lymphocytes in the blood. Heterophil antibodies are detected by the rapid latex haemagglutination (monospot) test, which is positive in 90% of patients.

Treatment is supportive. Occasionally, if there is marked stertor, a dose of intravenous hydrocortisone is necessary. Antibiotics are indicated if secondary bacterial infection supervenes but amoxycillin should be avoided as it can cause a rash.

Lingual tonsillitis

This is an uncommon localised inflammation of the lingual tonsils and usually only becomes apparent after a standard tonsillectomy. The history is of repeated episodes of soreness and discomfort deep in the throat, often combined with malaise. The lingual tonsils will look enlarged and inflamed and there may be associated lymphadenopathy. Treatment of the acute attacks is symptomatic, combined with antibiotics. Surgery is difficult as lingual tonsils do not have a capsule, but, if indicated, is best performed using the KTP laser, thus reducing the risk of haemorrhage.

Fungal infections

Candida infection of the oral cavity, larynx and pharynx is not uncommon, especially in seriously ill and debilitated patients. It is a complication of radiotherapy to the head and neck and may be found under dentures that have not been adequately cleaned. Asthmatic patients taking steroid inhalers may develop infection with candida. Fungal infection is the most common cause of failure with tracheo-oesophageal voice prostheses.

Patients with 'thrush' are generally asymptomatic, apart from slight soreness and bleeding caused by associated inflammation. Infection of the oesophagus with candida may cause marked odynophagia. On examination, white patches will be seen, which can be easily scraped off the mucous membrane.

Treatment is of the underlying disease or problem causing the infection. Antibiotics should be stopped if appropriate and topical nystatin suspension prescribed. If the infection is severe, a systemic antifungal agent such as fluconazole may be prescribed.

Diphtheria

This disease has virtually disappeared in most countries owing to an effective immunisation programme, but some parts of the world lack such preventative measures, and sporadic cases may also occur in developed countries. The disease is caused by *Corynebacterium diphtheriae*. It is disseminated by droplets (from coughing) and has an incubation period of up to 4 days. It mostly affects the fauces, and in moderate to severe cases a greyish membrane appears on the tonsils and pharyngeal wall. If severe, there can be gross oedema of the pharynx and stertorous breathing; the patient will be pyrexial and there may be superadded streptococcal infection.

A swab should be taken before treatment, which is with antitoxin and systemic penicillin. Complications include myocarditis and neuritis, and occasionally upper airway obstruction may be severe enough to warrant tracheostomy.

Agranulocytosis

Loss of neutrophils may be associated with ulcerative or necrotic pharyngeal or buccal lesions. Agranulocytosis may be idiopathic or secondary to drug administration; the spectrum of drugs that can cause agranulocytosis is wide, including many commonly administered ones (for example antibiotics such as chloramphenicol). Patients present with an irregular pyrexia and sore throat. Pharyngeal examination reveals superficial ulcers and a thin greyish membrane. A full blood count and film are diagnostic. Causative drugs are withdrawn and antibiotics are given in high doses. Haematological or immunological advice should be sought promptly for definitive management.

Tuberculosis

This is rare in the pharynx and is usually secondary to pulmonary tuberculosis. It presents as a deep ulcer, often involving the tonsil. It is easily mistaken for a carcinoma, emphasising the importance of biopsy of a presumed carcinoma prior to treatment. Investigation is by biopsy and chest X-ray and treatment is by the usual regimen of prolonged combination chemotherapy.

RETROPHARYNGEAL ABSCESS

This abscess is due to infection of retropharyngeal lymph nodes. It is dealt with fully in Chapter 18.

LARYNGITIS

Acute laryngitis

Acute laryngitis usually occurs as part of a generalised upper respiratory tract infection, often following on from a common cold. It is most frequently caused by adenoviruses or influenza viruses but secondary bacterial infection may supervene. Smoking and alcohol abuse as well as exposure to fumes at work predispose to acute laryngitis. It tends to be more problematical in people who use their voice professionally, such as teachers and singers, probably because they are unable to rest the voice sufficiently when they have an attack. It is also most common in those with coexistent nasal disease. The pathology is that of an acute inflammatory response.

Symptoms vary, depending upon the severity of the attack. The main symptoms are hoarseness, discomfort and pain in the larynx and often an irritating cough. The voice is weak and husky and gets worse during the day but is usually not lost completely. There may be associated 'flu like symptoms. Examination may reveal a pharyngitis. If indirect laryngoscopy is performed the larynx will be red and swollen, with the true cords being thickened and rounded; the whole larynx may be covered with mucus.

Treatment is symptomatic. The condition usually runs a short course with complete resolution. Voice rest is essential, along with humidification by steam inhalation and avoidance of irritants. Paracetamol or aspirin gargles may be soothing. If there is evidence of superadded bacterial infection, an antibiotic such as amoxycillin should be prescribed. Recurrent acute laryngitis with incomplete resolution may predispose to chronic laryngitis.

Supraglottitis (epiglottitis)

For a full description of acute epiglottitis in children, see Chapter 28. In adults, supraglottitis is a less fulminating disease; the larynx is proportionately larger and laryngeal oedema is not as dangerous. The microbiology is more diverse than in children and streptococcal infections are more common. The patient is unwell, with hoarseness, a severe sore throat and varying degrees of stridor. Indirect or fibreoptic laryngoscopy can be carried out safely in adults but facilities for emergency intubation or tracheostomy should be readily available. A red, swollen epiglottis is seen, with associated laryngeal and pharyngeal oedema.

Patients can usually be managed successfully with intravenous broad-spectrum antibiotics and intravenous steroids. Tracheostomy or intubation for 48 hours may be necessary. Once the infection has settled, the larynx should be examined to exclude an underlying malignancy.

Chronic laryngitis

This condition includes several entities in which the laryngeal mucosa undergoes irreversible inflammatory change. While not always due to chronic infection, it is considered here for the sake of completeness. The predominant symptom is of persistent hoarseness and for this reason the diagnosis should not be made until a laryngeal carcinoma is excluded.

The most common cause is repeated acute laryngitis that does not resolve; most patients are smokers or exposed to fumes at work. There may be associated nasal or oral disease and gastro-oesophageal reflux has been associated with chronic laryngitis. Prolonged use of steroid inhalers can cause chronic hoarseness of the voice, which is reversed on stopping the use of the inhalers. Oedema is replaced by fibrosis and hyperplasia of the mucous membrane, resulting in thickening of the mucosa.

Examination reveals a reddened thickened larynx. The inflammation may be localised to one or both true or false cords but is usually bilateral, and there may be mucus stuck to the larynx. The main symptom is hoarseness: the voice loses power during the course of the day and there may be an associated cough. The symptoms are very similar to those produced by laryngeal carcinoma, so anyone with a hoarse voice for more than 2 weeks should be referred for indirect laryngoscopy. In patients over 40 who are smokers, the diagnosis is carcinoma of the larynx until proved otherwise.

The treatment is to exclude predisposing factors, for example smoking and exposure to fumes, and to treat nasal disease if necessary. If the signs in the larynx are predominantly unilateral, a microlaryngoscopy is indicated, with biopsies to exclude carcinoma. Symptomatic measures, as described for acute laryngitis, are recommended and referral to a speech therapist may be helpful. Surgical debulking of florid inflamed mucosa, either by stripping or by laser vaporisation, should be considered only after these conservative measures have been tried.

Tuberculosis

Laryngeal tuberculosis is a complication of pulmonary tuberculosis except on the rarest of occasions. It is by no means uncommon in certain parts of the world and should always be considered in the differential diagnoses of laryngeal carcinoma. Direct implantation in the larynx of infected sputum is the most usual method of infection and the tendency is for healing as the chest condition improves.

Usually the patient is already known to be suffering from pulmonary tuberculosis. Hoarseness occurs and may be intermittent to start with. Pain on swallowing and speaking develops as ulceration becomes more marked.

Classically tuberculosis affects the posterior commisure and arytenoids but may involve one or both cords; the mucosa is red and swollen but may become ulcerated. Diagnosis is by a high index of suspicion, biopsy, chest X-ray and sputum examination. Treatment is as for pulmonary tuberculosis.

Perichondritis

This disorder is a chronic deep-seated infection of the laryngeal skeleton, caused by radiotherapy to a carcinoma, the tumour itself or, very rarely, tuberculosis or syphilis. The condition manifests with severe pain on swallowing and talking (opiates may be necessary to relieve the pain), as well as swelling and tenderness over the affected cartilage. Laryngeal oedema may cause airway obstruction.

Treatment consists of prolonged high dose antibiotic therapy. If available, hyperbaric oxygen therapy may be used as a supplementary treatment to antibiotics. A tracheostomy may be necessary for airway obstruction. If antibiotic therapy is unsuccessful and the pain persists, a laryngectomy is indicated. Although a somewhat drastic step, the diseased larynx is useless and the patient will be able to swallow painlessly and speak with the aid of modern voice restoration techniques.

> **Key points**
>
> ➤ Pharyngitis may be secondary to irritants, either endogenous or exogenous, e.g. cigarette smoke.
> ➤ Acute pharyngitis is usually streptococcal and occurs in outbreaks.
> ➤ Treatment of pharyngitis is by removing the irritant and simple symptomatic measures.
> ➤ Always perform a full blood count in cases of pharyngeal ulceration.
> ➤ Chronic pharyngeal ulcers are not always neoplastic.
> ➤ Retropharyngeal abscesses can lead to airway obstruction and mediastinitis and need to be treated very aggressively.
> ➤ Never ascribe persistent hoarseness to chronic laryngitis until a carcinoma has been excluded.

Paediatric airway disease

STRIDOR

Stridor is the most common manifestation of paediatric airway disease. It is the audible result of turbulent airflow in the larynx or trachea. Its phase during the respiratory cycle and its characteristics can help locate the site of an obstruction. Supraglottic stridor is classically inspiratory, glottic or subglottic stridor biphasic; and tracheal stridor expiratory. Stridor must be distinguished from stertor, which is generated by pharyngeal obstruction.

History

In acute airway obstruction, examination and resuscitation of the child should take place concurrently while obtaining the history of the episode from the parents. Foreign body ingestion should be excluded and symptoms of generalised illness noted.

In the more chronic situation a full paediatric history should be obtained, while at the same time taking note of the child's breathing. The obstetric and perinatal history is important, as premature infants may have been intubated for ventilation and this can result in complications in the airway. Onset of symptoms at birth suggests a fixed congenital narrowing; dynamic conditions, such as laryngomalacia and vocal fold paralysis, present in the early weeks but airway haemangiomas classically not before 6 weeks of age. Progressive stridor is typical of airway haemangiomas but may also be due to extrinsic tracheal compression by a mediastinal mass. Other symptoms, such as hoarseness, cough and apnoeic episodes, should be noted. Feeding difficulties, including regurgitation and aspiration, frequently accompany chronic airway obstruction in children. The increased respiratory effort required in the presence of a compromised airway combined with feeding problems may result in failure to thrive. Systematic questioning about other symptoms is important; for example, vocal fold paralysis may be associated with neurological disease, congenital cardiac anomalies or the corrective surgery thereof.

Examination

It is essential to assess the severity of the airway obstruction while searching for the cause. The degree of tracheal tug and intercostal recession will increase with increased respiratory effort and reduced airway diameter. Cyanosis is a late sign and is often associated with exhaustion of the child rather than worsening of the airway. In the acute situation, when a child's airway is seriously compromised, intervention to secure the airway may be necessary prior to further investigation.

Investigation of persistent stridor

The gold standard investigation to establish the cause of persistent stridor is microlaryngoscopy and bronchoscopy under general anaesthesia. Flexible fibreoptic laryngoscopy as an outpatient procedure may be useful in the diagnosis of glottic or supra-

187

glottic pathology, especially the dynamic disorders such as laryngomalacia and vocal fold paralysis, but even if a diagnosis is made using this technique, it should be remembered that 5% of patients will have dual pathology in the airway. Other investigations which may be useful include a chest X-ray, penetrated views of the larynx and tracheobronchial tree, bronchography, videofluoroscopy, CT and MRI of the airway, echocardiography to examine the anatomy of the heart and great vessels and laryngeal ultrasonography for vocal fold mobility. Investigation for gastro-oesophageal reflux may also be relevant. Common causes of airway obstruction in infants are listed in Table 28.1.

Acute epiglottitis

This is a life-threatening condition and should be treated in hospital. It is usually due to *Haemophilus influenzae* infection. The epiglottis swells rapidly and any attempt to examine the throat may induce fatal laryngeal obstruction. A slight sore throat or upper respiratory infection may precede the rapid onset of severe symptoms. Dysphagia occurs early and a change in cry or voice is characteristic. Inspiratory stridor develops rapidly and may progress, if untreated, to fatal obstruction within a few hours.

Other causes of acute stridor and dysphagia, such as foreign body ingestion, diphtheria and retropharyngeal abscess, must be excluded. A lateral radiograph of the neck may assist in the differential diagnosis but it may not be safe to perform this in

Table 28.1 Causes of airway obstruction in children

Site	Pathology
Supralaryngeal	Pierre Robin sequence
	Craniofacial malformations
	Cystic hygroma
Supraglottic	Laryngomalacia
Glottic	Vocal fold paralysis
	Glottic web
Subglottic	Subglottic stenosis
	Subglottic cyst
	Haemangioma
Transglottic	Cleft larynx

the seriously ill child. Direct examination of the larynx is diagnostic but must be delayed until facilities for intubation and tracheostomy are available. Intubation is preferable, as the illness only lasts a few days, but ultimately the choice of airway management depends on the anaesthetic, surgical and nursing skills available. Medical treatment with fluids and appropriate intravenous antibiotics follows once the airway has been secured.

Acute laryngotracheobronchitis

This is less dangerous than acute epiglottitis but the severity should not be underestimated. Following an upper respiratory tract infection, a child may develop marked inspiratory stridor with a high pyrexia and toxaemia. The stridor is due to oedema, initially subglottic then spreading down the tracheobronchial tree. Sticky secretions form crusts, which may be a serious cause of obstruction and difficult to remove. The aetiology is viral. Medical treatment with nebulised adrenaline, inhaled or intravenous steroids and humidification may be successful but, if not, intubation or tracheostomy will be necessary to secure the airway.

Laryngomalacia

Laryngomalacia is responsible for more than two-thirds of congenital stridor cases. The stridor is classically inspiratory, worse when the baby is active and relieved by a prone posture. It usually increases in severity over the first few months of life and then starts to resolve spontaneously. Diagnosis may be made at endoscopy with the child breathing spontaneously. Classical appearances described include an omega-shaped epiglottis, short aryepiglottic folds and loose, redundant mucosa over the arytenoid cartilages. On inspiration the cartilages are sucked inwards, obstructing the airway (Fig. 28.1). In more than 90% of cases no further intervention is necessary once the diagnosis has been established. Parental reassurance and regular review to ensure complete resolution of symptoms is enough. In severe laryngomalacia, persistent respiratory distress and associated feeding difficulties due to gastro-oesophageal reflux may result in failure to thrive. Aryepiglottoplasty including division of the aryepiglottic folds and excision of the redundant mucosa has largely replaced tracheostomy in the management of such patients.

Vocal fold paralysis

Vocal fold paralysis is rare in children but is nevertheless an important cause of neonatal stridor. Bilateral paralysis usually presents with stridor, cyanosis and apnoea, and unilateral paralysis more subtly with dysphonia; the latter is said to occur less frequently but this may be a failure of diagnosis. Feeding problems are equally common in the two groups.

The diagnosis is established at endoscopy: one or both cords may be observed to be fixed in a median or paramedian position. Paradoxical inspiratory adduction of the cords sometimes occurs but attention to diaphragmatic movements to determine the inspiratory and expiratory phases of respiration will reveal this. Rigid endoscopy under general anaesthesia with the patient breathing spontaneously is preferable to flexible fibreoptic laryngoscopy, as it permits palpation of the vocal folds to distinguish true paralysis from cricoarytenoid joint fixation. It also permits observation of vocal fold mobility even in the presence of laryngomalacia.

Management depends on symptom severity and a knowledge of the aetiology and likelihood of recovery. The airway should be secured by intubation or tracheostomy if symptoms are severe or progressive; it may be necessary in up to a third of unilateral cases and 75% of bilateral cases.

Vocal fold paralysis in children may be due to neurological disease, meningomyelocele with Arnold–Chiari malformation and hydrocephalus, birth trauma and surgical trauma, particularly tracheo-oesophageal fistula repair and correction of congenital cardiac anomalies. Central lesions are more frequently associated with bilateral paralysis, and peripheral lesions with a unilateral problem. In up to a third of children vocal fold paralysis is said to be idiopathic, these children often have other congenital anomalies, mainly pulmonary, cardiovascular and oesophageal.

Spontaneous recovery of vocal fold paralysis is unpredictable in children. The value of electromyography in establishing prognosis is uncertain. If recovery is going to occur, it is usually within 6 months; late recovery has been reported but may be complicated by laryngeal muscle atrophy, synkinesis and cricoarytenoid joint fixation. Early recovery is more likely in acquired than congenital paralysis and in unilateral than bilateral cases.

Infants with unilateral vocal fold paralysis requiring tracheostomy can usually be decannulated by the age of 2, even if the paralysis persists. Any persistent dysphonia usually responds to voice therapy, although medialisation procedures may be necessary; the latter may also improve aspiration. In bilateral paralysis, cord lateralisation may permit decannulation if spontaneous recovery does not occur. An improvement in the airway is usually at the expense of voice quality and may exacerbate any tendency to aspiration. Alternatively, successful reinnervation of the posterior cricoarytenoid muscles may permit decannulation without complications; it is only suitable in selected cases. Irreversible surgical decisions should where possible be delayed until negligible hope of spontaneous recovery of function remains and, preferably, until the child is old enough to take part in such decisions.

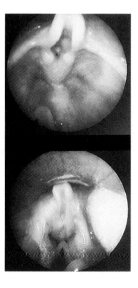

Fig. 28.1 Laryngomalacia. Larynx obstructed by inwards collapse of cartilages on inspiration. Note omega-shaped epiglottis.

Airway haemangiomas

These capillary haemangiomas occur most frequently in the subglottis and are usually solitary but may be multiple. In 50% of cases they are associated with cervicofacial cutaneous haemangiomas. Presentation is with stridor at about 6 weeks of age, often initially intermittent and misdiagnosed as croup, but gradually progressive as the haemangioma enlarges. The stridor is exacerbated by crying or upper respiratory infections. The appearance of airway haemangiomas is pathognomonic and diagnosis can be made at direct laryngoscopy: biopsy is not usually necessary.

The natural history of the lesion is rapid proliferation up to the age of 1 year and then spontaneous involution, which, together with the growth of the larynx, allows resolution of airway symptoms by 2–3 years of age. Active management to secure the airway may be necessary in over 50% of cases. Tracheostomy will bypass the lesion and may be necessary for up to 2 years. Various interventions, both local and systemic, have been employed to hasten involution of the lesion, shorten the period of cannulation or obviate the need for tracheostomy.

Radiotherapy is effective but carries unacceptable side-effects for this benign condition in infants. Local treatments with cryotherapy, sclerosants and the carbon dioxide laser are all associated with subglottic stenosis. Systemic treatment with corticosteroids is effective in most cases, but treatment may be required for up to 18 months and carries a significant risk of associated complications. Systemic interferon α_{2a} also accelerates regression of haemangiomas but side-effects, including bone marrow suppression and neurotoxicity, may preclude long-term treatment. Successful management using intralesional corticosteroid injections followed by prolonged intubation has been reported to avoid tracheostomy in some cases. Submucous resection of the lesion via a laryngofissure can be complicated by subglottic stenosis and it may be more effective if combined with a subglottic expansion procedure. It appears to be regaining popularity.

Laryngotracheal stenosis

This may be congenital or acquired. Stenosis most frequently affects the subglottis (Fig. 28.2), the

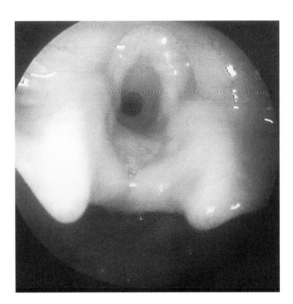

Fig. 28.2 Subglottic stenosis.

narrowest part of the airway and the only part surrounded by a complete ring of cartilage, the cricoid, which limits its lumen. Causes of stenosis include internal trauma from heat inhalation, caustic ingestion or endotracheal intubation – the most common aetiology (Box 28.1) – and external trauma from sharp or blunt injuries or high tracheostomy.

Presentation depends on the severity of the stenosis (Table 28.2) and varies from intermittent stridor with upper respiratory tract infections to persistent stridor and dyspnoea. Patients may also present when extubation of an endotracheal tube 'fails'. Extubation may be facilitated by conservative measures, including steroids, antireflux treatment and nebulised adrenaline. If these fail, a cricoid split may be successful.

Mild to moderate stenosis, often congenital, can sometimes be managed expectantly, waiting for growth of the larynx to expand the subglottis. More severe stenosis may necessitate tracheostomy to secure the airway, although this results in bacterial contamination of the larynx and may exacerbate inflammatory changes and later scar formation.

Laryngotracheal reconstruction to enlarge the lumen of the stenotic segment of the airway is the most successful approach to treatment of established stenosis. The cartilaginous framework is split anteriorly

Pathogenesis of subglottic stenosis following endotracheal intubation

- ■ Patient factors
  - – Shape and size of larynx
  - – Gastro-oesophageal reflux
  - – Sepsis
  - – Activity of patient
  - – General debility
  - – Dehydration
- ■ Extrinsic factors
  - – Traumatic intubation
  - – Multiple intubations
  - – Movement of endotracheal tube
  - – Endotracheal tube shape
  - – Endotracheal tube composition
  - – Sterilisation technique
  - – Endotracheal tube size
  - – Duration of intubation
  - – Subsequent tracheostomy

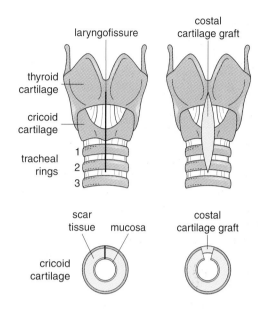

Fig. 28.3 Technique of laryngotracheal reconstruction. Anterior view of larynx (above) and transverse section of subglottis (below), before (left) and after (right) insertion of the shaped costal cartilage graft.

and/or posteriorly, via a laryngofissure. The circumference is then augmented with grafts, usually of costal cartilage (Fig. 28.3). This is followed by a period of stenting to stabilise the reconstruction and prevent restenosis. This can be performed (1) as a primary procedure, rather than tracheostomy, allowing extubation a few days later – single stage laryngotracheal reconstruction; or (2) as a delayed step, after tracheostomy in the management of more severe stenosis. Cricotracheal resection of the stenotic segment with end-to-end anastomosis is suitable only for a short stenosis separate from the glottis.

Table 28.2 Grading system for subglottic stenosis based on assessment of the percentage of obstruction

Grade	Obstruction (%)
1	0–50
2	51–70
3	71–99
4	100

RECURRENT RESPIRATORY PAPILLOMATOSIS

Recurrent respiratory papillomatosis is due to epithelial infection with human papilloma virus types 6 or 11; the latter is associated with more severe disease. It is characterised by single or multiple benign, non-keratinising squamous papillomas. It usually affects the larynx, presenting with gradually increasing hoarseness or stridor but, in severe disease, may affect the entire respiratory tract including the tracheobronchial tree (25%) and, rarely, the pulmonary parenchyma (less than 1%). Recurrent respiratory papillomatosis presents more frequently in children than in adults, the peak incidence occurring between 2 and 5 years of age. Management is directed towards maintenance of the airway, with avoidance of tracheostomy, and preservation of voice. Because clinically normal respiratory epithelium is infected, mechanical removal of papillomas cannot effect a cure. Remission may occur spontaneously but early onset and severe disease make it less likely; it is not associated with the onset of puberty, as has previously been suggested. Relapse may be precipitated by trauma or immunosuppression.

Endoscopic carbon dioxide laser vaporisation of

lesions, repeated as necessary, is the management of choice for the airway. Complications do occur, related to the frequency of surgery, and include vocal fold fibrosis, web formation at the anterior and posterior commissures of the glottis, interarytenoid scarring and arytenoid fixation, and laryngeal stenosis. These can be minimised by attention to laser emission parameters, depth of vaporisation and surgical technique, sparing the anterior commissure; debulking rather than total extirpation of lesions is recommended. The KTP laser is preferred for lesions in the trachea and bronchial tree.

Tracheostomy may be necessary to secure the airway in severe cases. The presence of a tracheostomy is associated with an increased risk of tracheal and pulmonary papillomatosis. The latter is an uncommon but progressive complication; it carries a 50% mortality from cardiorespiratory failure. Malignant degeneration to laryngotracheal carcinoma or squamous cell carcinoma of the bronchus is rare but has been reported.

Effective systemic adjuvant therapy has been sought. Ribavirin, a broad-spectrum antiviral agent, causes significant regression of papillomas but is teratogenic in rodents. Human leucocyte interferon may induce partial or complete remission but there is a rebound effect on cessation of treatment and no increase in prolonged remissions.

Effective future management will probably be directed towards prevention of infection. It is likely that children become infected either in utero or intrapartum from maternal genital papillomas in some cases, but transmissibility is low and may be further reduced by maternal treatment during gestation and delivery by caesarean section.

PAEDIATRIC TRACHEOSTOMY

The general indications for tracheostomy in infants and children are to relieve airway obstruction, to facilitate mechanical ventilation or to reduce the dead space and improve the management of secretions in chronic lung disease. The introduction of diphtheria antitoxin, followed by the active immunisation programmes for diphtheria and polio, together with the development of endotracheal intubation as preferred primary airway management in these conditions have significantly reduced

the frequency of paediatric tracheostomy over the last 100 years. More than 50% of paediatric tracheostomies are now performed in infants less than 1 year old, usually for congenital problems or for acquired subglottic stenosis, a complication of frequent or prolonged endotracheal intubation in some preterm infants. Airway trauma or infection are more likely to precipitate tracheostomy in the older child.

Technique

Paediatric tracheostomy is performed under general anaesthesia with endotracheal intubation, the patient in a supine position. The neck should be extended but not overextended as this will draw the thoracic structures (including pleura, mediastinal vessels and the thymus) up into the neck and increase the risk of complications. A 1–2 cm horizontal skin crease incision midway between the cricoid and the suprasternal notch is planned and the skin infiltrated with local anaesthesia. A tracheostomy tube of appropriate length and diameter for the child is selected and checked; its connections should conform with standard anaesthetic circuits.

After the skin incision, the trachea is identified by palpation; a combination of sharp and blunt dissection or bipolar diathermy dissection can be used, keeping to the midline between the strap muscles and through the thyroid isthmus until the trachea is identified visually. Non-absorbable stay sutures are positioned bilaterally through the second and third or third and fourth rings of tracheal cartilage and haemostasis is ensured. After warning the anaesthetist, a vertical tracheotomy is performed between the stay sutures (Fig. 28.4). If the tracheotomy is too high, there is a risk of subsequent subglottic stenosis; if too low, there is a risk of the tracheostomy tube being diverted into the right main bronchus. Any secretions or blood in the airway are aspirated using suction and then the endotracheal tube gradually withdrawn by the anaesthetist so that the tip is in the subglottis while the tracheostomy tube is introduced into the trachea. If there is any difficulty with insertion, the endotracheal tube can be advanced back down the trachea. After the tube is sited, the anaesthetic circuit is reconnected, the wound closed loosely around the tube and the tube secured in

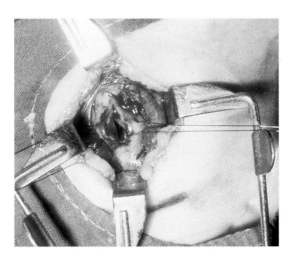

Fig. 28.4 Paediatric tracheostomy. Note the stay sutures securing the edges of the incised trachea.

position with tapes, with the neck in flexion. The stay sutures are taped to the skin; their purpose is to facilitate the first tube change, or recannulation if decannulation occurs accidentally before the tract has become established.

Postoperatively a chest radiograph is routinely checked to establish the level of the tip of the tracheostomy tube. If it is abutting the carina or in the right main bronchus it should be withdrawn slightly, or changed for a shorter tube. Ideally, the child should be cared for by a paediatric nurse experienced in tracheostomy care: humidified air should be administered and regular suction of secretions performed. The first tube change is undertaken by the surgeon after 1 week and the stay sutures can then be removed.

Complications

Early complications of paediatric tracheostomy are the same as those of adult tracheostomy: haemorrhage, pneumothorax, surgical emphysema, infection, tube obstruction, accidental decannulation and creation of a false passage; however, the risk of damaging intrathoracic structures is higher than in the adult, especially for the inexperienced surgeon. Tube obstruction, which in adults is usually the result of secretions, can also be caused in young babies by the soft tissue below the chin; this can be managed by

appropriate adaptation of the tracheostomy tube.

Tube obstruction and accidental decannulation continue to be risks in the long term and are more dangerous the more severe the airway obstruction above the tracheostomy. Other delayed complications include granulation tissue caused by the presence of the tube, either superficially on the skin or in the trachea, suprastomally or at tube tip level. Bleeding, tube obstruction and difficulty in changing the tube may result. Suprastomal collapse and laryngotracheal stenosis can also occur. Children with tracheostomies are at increased risk of chest infection; this may be related to frequent tracheal suction or to silent aspiration, the latter being common in the presence of a tracheostomy.

Mortality rates in paediatric tracheostomy vary in different institutions and different countries, depending on referral patterns and social circumstances, but rates as low as 1–2% should be achievable. Death is usually the result of tube obstruction or displacement and is more likely if the airway obstruction above the tube is complete.

Delay in the development of speech and language occurs in infants with tracheostomies; sign language may facilitate communication. Even after decannulation, therapy will be required to improve breath control and assist a child to 'catch up'.

Behavioural problems have been reported in children with tracheostomies, both those institutionalised because of inadequate social circumstances and those cared for at home. Parental anxiety, communication difficulties and frequent hospital admissions may contribute in the latter group of children. Home care for children with long-term tracheostomies should be encouraged where possible: parental education in suction techniques, tube changing and cardiopulmonary resuscitation should precede the child's discharge from hospital and the necessary equipment must be provided at home. Support for the parents from the specialist centre performing the tracheostomy should always be available, including emergency medical care, speech and language therapy and social support where necessary. Regular endoscopy every 6–12 months will allow evaluation and management of any complications, as well as reassessment of the underlying pathology and the need for tracheostomy.

Tracheostomy tubes

A variety of tracheostomy tubes is available for children. The ideal tube should optimise airflow by having a short shaft, a maximum radius of curvature and a smooth inner surface. It should be comfortable, easy to clean, easy to change, with standard attachments (e.g. for speaking valves or anaesthetic circuits), cosmetically acceptable, and, ideally, inexpensive. Multiple widths and lengths should be available for children of different ages, and tubes increased in size as a child grows.

Metal tubes, although expensive, are reusable and will last for many years. Their rigidity means that they have the maximum internal diameter for their external diameter. They usually have an inner and an outer tube so that they are easy to unblock in an emergency, simply by removal of the inner tube. However, they have largely been superseded by synthetic tubes, which seem to be more cosmetically acceptable. Synthetic tubes are generally thicker walled with no inner tube. It is said that their thermoplastic properties allow them to conform to a patient's anatomy, reducing the risk of ulceration and granulations. Each tube is relatively inexpensive but they are not reusable and usually need changing every 1–2 weeks. Fenestrated tracheostomy tubes are not commonly used in children; if air can escape through the larynx around the tube a speaking valve can be used to allow phonation. Some children prefer to use a finger to close the tube for phonation but this is less hygienic: others unconsciously learn to use chin dipping for the same purpose.

Decannulation

Before any attempt at decannulation, microlaryngoscopy and bronchoscopy should be undertaken to ensure that there has been resolution of the original lesion and that no complications are present which might compromise success, such as granulations, suprastomal collapse or subglottic stenosis. If all is well, ward decannulation can be planned, in which the tube is progressively reduced in size, then blocked for 24 hours and, finally, removed. Throughout this process, which may take several days, the child's general well-being, respiratory rate and oxygenation are monitored and, if adversely affected, the process can be reversed at any stage, reverting to a full-sized tracheostomy tube for the child's age.

If there is significant suprastomal collapse, surgical decannulation may be necessary: under general anaesthesia with nasotracheal intubation the tracheostomy tube is removed, the skin stoma and tract excised and the tracheal stoma formally closed in layers. The child can usually be extubated within 48 hours. In mild subglottic stenosis, the tracheal circumference can be augmented with a cartilage graft at the time of surgical decannulation.

Tracheocutaneous fistula

The incidence of this complication of decannulation increases with the length of time that the tracheostomy has been present; it may occur in up to 50% of ward decannulations. It is easily managed by surgical closure if it persists for more than 6 months.

GASTRO-OESOPHAGEAL REFLUX DISEASE

This is defined as any symptomatic condition or histopathological alteration resulting from episodes of gastro-oesophageal reflux. Gastro-oesophageal reflux is prevalent in normal newborn infants but predisposing factors include preterm delivery, laryngomalacia, intubation, recumbency and the presence of a gastrostomy, all common features encountered in paediatric otolaryngology. The usual manifestations are oesophageal, most frequently simply regurgitation and vomiting but sometimes complicated by anaemia, haematemesis and melaena, dysphagia and failure to thrive. Atypical presentations of gastro-oesophageal reflux include laryngeal and pulmonary manifestations, such as laryngospasm, subglottic stenosis and apnoeas. The pathology of gastro-oesophageal reflux disease may be a result of the direct effect of gastric acid, bile salts or enzymes on mucosa or to reflex effects mediated by the vagus. Investigations to assess severity include barium oesophagography, oesophageal pH monitoring, endoscopy and oesophageal biopsy.

Mild disease can be managed by parental reassurance and thickening feeds. If symptoms persist, prokinetic agents will improve peristalsis, increase the lower oesophageal sphincter pressure and improve gastric emptying. Histamine receptor (type 2) antagonists may be added if there is oesophagitis. For refractory cases a proton pump inhibitor may be necessary. Surgical management is reserved for patients with a predisposing anatomical anomaly, such as diaphragmatic hernia or gastric outlet obstruction, or if an oesophageal stricture has developed. The Nissen fundoplication procedure is recommended after failure of medical treatment; it is effective in 90% of cases.

FOREIGN BODIES

Foreign body inhalation is not infrequent in children between the ages of 1 and 3 years, twice as commonly in boys as in girls. Objects likely to be inhaled include nuts and seeds and small pieces of toys. Larger objects may impact in the larynx; smaller ones pass through it down the trachea and generally lodge in the right main bronchus, as it is wider than the left and the interbronchial septum projects to the left.

A foreign body in the larynx may present with acute respiratory distress but in the lower airway the symptoms and signs are more subtle. There is usually an initial history of choking or coughing and this may be followed by a persistent wheeze. However, there may be no further symptoms after the initial event and this can lead to a delay in diagnosis. Persistent or recurrent lobar pneumonia should lead to suspicion of a foreign body in the airway.

Acute respiratory distress necessitates urgent intervention. If time allows, examination may direct the clinician to the site of the foreign body – hoarseness, stridor and excessive salivation suggest a laryngeal foreign body; unilateral expiratory wheeze and reduced air entry may indicate a foreign body in the bronchus. The presence of the foreign body may cause an inflammatory reaction of the bronchial mucosa and the production of granulation tissue, particularly if it is of vegetable origin. Obstruction of the bronchial lumen results in distal atelectasis, which may progress to lobar pneumonia or a lung abscess.

Radiological examination of the airway, including inspiratory, expiratory and lateral chest radiographs, may assist in diagnosis, revealing any radio-opaque foreign body, mediastinal shift as a result of obstructive emphysema or atelectasis, and collapse or consolidation of the lung. The latter changes are unlikely to be present within 24 hours of inhalation.

Suspected foreign body inhalation is an indication for early endoscopy under general anaesthesia by personnel experienced in paediatric airway management. A laryngeal foreign body may be removed at direct laryngoscopy; tracheal and bronchial foreign bodies by using a rigid bronchoscope and grasping forceps. If granulation tissue has developed, the application of a 10% adrenaline solution will minimise bleeding and improve access. In the rare situation where endoscopic retrieval of a foreign body is unsuccessful, it may be necessary to proceed to thoracotomy and bronchotomy.

Following successful extraction of a foreign body, it is important to have a second look to ensure that there are no remaining fragments, particularly in the case of vegetable matter. The bronchial tree distal to the foreign body should also be aspirated to hasten resolution of atelectasis or infection. Postoperative antibiotics and physiotherapy may be beneficial in selected cases.

> ### ➤ Key points
>
> - ➤ In children with stridor, resuscitation, history and examination should take place concurrently.
> - ➤ Do not attempt to examine the throat if acute epiglottitis is suspected.
> - ➤ Laryngomalacia is the most common cause of congenital stridor.
> - ➤ Suspicion of an inhaled foreign body is an indication for early endoscopy.

Non-neoplastic disease of the larynx and pharynx

29

INFLAMMATORY LARYNGEAL LESIONS

Several different types of inflammatory lesion of the larynx are recognised (Fig. 29.1).

Contact ulcer

Thickening and heaping up of the mucous membrane may be found in areas of the larynx subjected to trauma or excessive abnormal movement. There is a change in the quality of voice, sometimes amounting to true hoarseness. This hypertrophic change may be localised to the area of the vocal process of the arytenoids and produce the condition of 'contact ulcer', where the thickened area on one cord impinges on the other, giving the appearance of an ulcer, although in fact the epithelium is intact. Biopsy is needed to exclude malignancy (such patients are often heavy smokers). Treatment aims to restore normal laryngeal function, which is achieved by stopping smoking, referral for intensive speech therapy and endoscopic excision of hypertrophic tissue. Gastro-oesophageal reflux is thought to be at least a contributory factor in the pathogenesis of this condition and should be treated if present.

Vocal nodules (Singer's nodes)

These occur at the area of maximum vibration of the vocal cords, namely at the junction of the anterior third and posterior two-thirds of the cord (halfway along the membranous cord). The nodules are by definition bilateral and present as localised hard thickenings on the edge of each cord. The abnormality is submucosal (of fibrosis following acute inflammation) so the mucosa appears normal. This condition is caused by misuse of the voice and bad voice production, often in the presence of inflammation, and is common in schoolchildren ('screamers' nodes') as well as actors, teachers and singers who have not undergone formal voice training.

Non-surgical treatment is often successful. Voice rest, removal of any inflammatory focus and speech therapy often lead to resorption of the nodules and restoration of a normal voice; if not, precise localised removal is curative.

Intubation granuloma

This is a rare consequence of endotracheal intubation, usually occurring after a traumatic intubation. Patients are referred a few days or weeks after an operation with a very hoarse voice; there is rarely stridor. Indirect laryngoscopy reveals a large fleshy granuloma arising from one arytenoid; this can be removed endoscopically, preferably with the laser to aid haemostasis. The differential diagnosis of prolonged hoarseness after intubation is arytenoid dislocation; relocation to its correct position is possible in the early stages but thereafter a permanent disability develops because of fibrosis.

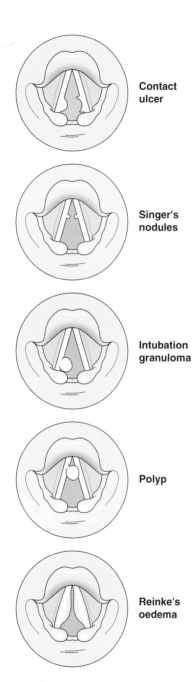

Contact ulcer

Singer's nodules

Intubation granuloma

Polyp

Reinke's oedema

Fig. 29.1 Inflammatory lesions of the vocal cords.

Vocal polyp

Polyps can occur in several different areas of the larynx but are most often seen attached to the vocal cords. A polyp appears as a smooth glistening body attached to one cord; it may have a pedicle or it may be sessile, and the size of the polyp can vary enormously. It may be readily localised, or sometimes polypoidal change may affect the entire length of one or both vocal cords. Patients complain of long-standing hoarseness. Initially, a polyp may not be visible until the patient is asked to cough, when it will be seen to have arisen from the undersurface of the cord. Occasionally polyps can be so large that they cause stridor and airway obstruction; treatment is by laser debulking or by tracheostomy.

Definitive treatment is by precise endoscopic removal of the lesion. If the lesions are bilateral, stripping of the cords should be a staged procedure to prevent webbing at the anterior commissure. Removal of irritants to the larynx – such as cigarette smoke – and speech therapy are important parts of the treatment.

Laryngeal oedema (Reinke's oedema)

Increased volume of the contents in the subepithelial space beneath the vocal cords results in the characteristic swelling of the vocal cords called Reinke's oedema. It almost always occurs in smokers and results from smoking and voice abuse; it is most common in middle-aged women. The swelling is often considerable; it is invariably bilateral and may take on a polypoid appearance. Patients may appear hypothyroid but thyroid function tests are usually normal. Cessation of smoking and speech therapy are often unsuccessful on their own and staged stripping of both vocal cords is almost invariably required.

NEUROLOGICAL DISORDERS OF THE LARYNX

Sensory dysfunction

The sensory nerve supply to the supraglottis is from the vagus nerve via the internal laryngeal nerve. Stimulation produces a cough reflex which prevents food and saliva from entering the airway, thus being a very important protective reflex. Loss of this reflex predisposes to aspiration, which can be a very serious condition, especially in older patients with other neurological disorders. Uncontrolled aspiration leads to a severe pneumonia which is life threatening. In practice it may be appropriate not to actively treat patients with end-stage neurological disease, for example motor neurone disease. A pneumonia may provide a humane and painless means of death in such an intractable situation.

Sensory paralysis is caused by lesions affecting the vagus nerve in the skull base or the upper neck, or localised lesions involving the internal laryngeal nerve, the most common being iatrogenic after partial pharyngectomy. Aspiration almost invariably results, although this is usually temporary and these patients often tolerate moderate degrees of aspiration reasonably well.

The first principle of aspiration management is to protect the airway: tracheostomy with placement of a cuffed tracheostomy tube (with some form of fenestration to help with speech production) is effective. The epiglottis can be sutured to the aryepiglottic fold to protect the laryngeal inlet more comfortably (epiglottopexy). Thickened feeds and modified swallowing techniques may help prevent aspiration to a greater or lesser extent, while the help of an experienced speech and language therapist can be invaluable.

Laryngeal spasm

This is most commonly seen postoperatively in patients with a sensitive larynx that has been irritated by secretions or blood. The cords become adducted and the patient cannot breathe. This usually settles quickly with oxygen therapy but the patient may need to be reanaesthetised.

Laryngeal spasm may present in the clinic, with repeated choking episodes and loss of voice. The patient is very frightened but the experience is momentary and they are rarely cyanosed. It is thought that airway irritants such as gastro-oesophageal reflux or a postnasal drip, may be the cause and these should be looked for and treated if found.

'Functional dysphonia' is a form of laryngeal spasm which is often induced by anxiety or panic attacks; it is most common in young females who present with an aphonia. The vocal cords will be seen lying equidistant from the midline. They move normally on deep inspiration but on phonation will not meet in the midline. Patients are able to cough normally and when they do so, the cords will meet in the midline.

Treatment of functional dysphonia is of the underlying cause. Positive reassurance is required, as well as the services of a good speech therapist. Teaching the patient to cough, and transforming this gradually into phonation is helpful. Psychological help may be necessary and there may be recurrence, but in general the prognosis is good.

Vocal fold paralysis

Table 29.1 outlines the causes of a vocal fold paralysis.

A vocal cord may be paralysed by mechanical fixation of the arytenoid or vocalis muscle (usually by tumour) or by a nerve palsy. The paralysis may be unilateral or bilateral and the cords paralysed in abduction or adduction, the latter being by far the most common. Bilateral vocal cord palsies in an adducted position are rare but cause severe stridor and an emergency tracheostomy is usually indicated.

Table 29.1 Causes of vocal fold paralysis

Cause	%
Mechanical	
Fixation by tumour	
Arytenoid fixation	
Dislocation	
Rheumatoid arthritis	
Recurrent laryngeal nerve palsy	
Malignant disease	30
Lung carcinoma	
Thyroid carcinoma	
Oesophageal carcinoma	
Surgical trauma	30
Idiopathic	20
Non-surgical trauma	7
Central/neurological	5
Inflammatory	4
Miscellaneous	4

Non-neoplastic disease of the larynx and pharynx

The most common cause is after total thyroidectomy when a bilateral recurrent laryngeal nerve palsy may result from inadvertent trauma during surgery.

Surgical trauma still remains a significant cause of unilateral vocal cord palsy. This is in part a result of more technically demanding procedures, both in the field of skull base surgery and in cardiothoracic surgery, where procedures on the infant heart and ductus arteriosus may cause a vocal fold paralysis. Paralysis after thyroid surgery is less common than it was, however, because of the recognition on the part of surgeons that the recurrent laryngeal nerve needs to be positively identified before any excision is made. The most common cause of a vocal cord palsy is malignancy, and the most common causative malignancy is a bronchogenic carcinoma, almost exclusively occurring on the left side.

The recurrent laryngeal nerve may be affected superiorly when it is still included in the vagus, or lower down when it has separated from the vagus nerve. It will be recalled that on the left side the recurrent nerve leaves the vagus as the latter crosses the arch of the aorta. On the right side, the recurrent laryngeal nerve leaves the vagus nerve as it crosses the subclavian artery. Lesions causing a left vocal fold paralysis are much more common than on the right, owing to the longer intrathoracic course of the left recurrent laryngeal nerve. The aetiology is therefore to some extent an exercise in anatomy, and lesions may occur at various levels:

- Bulbar lesions. Vascular lesions, multiple sclerosis and tumours.
- Jugular foramen lesions. These are nearly always caused by tumours such as glomus jugulare tumours.
- Lesions in the course of the nerve.
- Tumours in the neck, e.g. chemodectoma.
- Goitre and thyroidectomy.
- Pericarditis, aortic aneurysm and surgery in the region of the aortic arch.
- Bronchogenic carcinoma.
- Oesophageal carcinoma and mediastinal metastases.
- Neurological causes, for example diabetic neuritis or mononeuritis.
- Idiopathic causes: often a postviral palsy. This is a diagnosis of exclusion and normal function may be restored with time.

Various eponymous rules have been expounded to explain the types of motor paralysis and why the cord may lie in a paramedian position or more laterally (the cadaveric position). Although it is an interesting exercise to try and predict from the position of the cord the site of the lesion that is causing the palsy, it has no clinical relevance and theories such as Semon's law need not be learnt.

Symptoms

The patient will present with a hoarse, breathy voice, usually of quite short duration, and may have symptoms related to the cause of the palsy (for example haemoptysis and dyspnoea). The voice sometimes improves slightly because the contralateral cord has compensated for the palsy. There may be mild dysphagia due to cricopharyngeal spasm.

Examination

The paralysis may be complete or incomplete. In the incomplete stage the paralysed cord lies near the midline, and there is no outward movement on inspiration. On phonation the active cord approaches the weakened cord, so that good apposition occurs and a satisfactory voice results. At this stage it is thought that some of the adductor muscles are still functioning.

In the complete stage the adductor muscles are also paralysed so that the affected cord lies further away from the midline and phonation becomes poorer. The arytenoid cartilage tends to fall forwards so that the cord appears shorter and at a lower level than its active neighbour. In some patients with good compensation by the active cord, it may be noted that the active cord will actually cross the midline during phonation (Fig. 29.2).

Investigation

Details of the investigation of a patient with a unilateral vocal fold paralysis are shown in Box 29.1. The strategy at each stage is to identify or exclude any of the causes mentioned. Only when an exhaustive search has been made can the diagnosis of an 'idiopathic' palsy be made (Fig. 29.3).

Treatment is directed to the cause, if possible. If

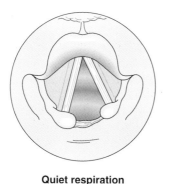 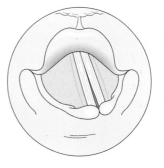

Quiet respiration   **Phonation**

Fig. 29.2 Paralysed left vocal cord on mirror examination during quiet respiration and phonation. The active cord can cross the midline and may succeed in closing the glottis to provide a good voice.

a patient is found to have a vocal cord palsy following thyroidectomy, the neck should be re-explored urgently as there may be a ligature involving the recurrent laryngeal nerve. A palsy secondary to a bronchogenic carcinoma indicates inoperability and carries a very poor prognosis.

The underlying problem causing a weak voice is a chink in the glottis on phonation, allowing air to escape. Thus the principle of treatment is to close the glottic chink, either by encouraging the active cord to compensate across the midline (speech therapy) or medialising the paralysed cord by some form of surgical procedure. Unless the patient is terminally ill, no surgical procedure should be undertaken for about 6 months after the palsy in

case spontaneous recovery occurs. Spontaneous recovery is more likely if the aetiology is viral.

The simplest way of medialising a vocal cord is by injecting some inert material lateral into the vocal cord to 'bulk up' these tissues, pushing the cord into the midline – Teflon paste or collagen may be used. This is simple and quick and indicated in ill patients who need a good voice for the rest of their lives, and involves only a brief anaesthetic. Teflon is injected endoscopically while collagen may be injected through the thyrohyoid membrane

---

■ Box 29.1

Investigation of a unilateral vocal fold paralysis

■ History
■ Examination including postnasal space and chest
■ Chest X-ray (CXR)
■ If CXR negative:
  – Panendoscopy, including oesophagoscopy and bronchoscopy and biopsy postnasal space
  – Sputum analysis for cytology
  – Fasting glucose, ESR, viral titres
  – CT of brainstem, skull base, neck to thorax down to bottom of aortic arch

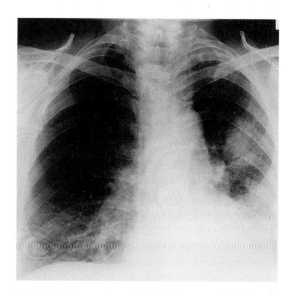

Fig. 29.3 A chest radiograph is the first investigation to be obtained in a patient with a paralysed vocal fold. A left-sided hilar mass is present.

under endoscopic guidance. Although rather imprecise, Teflon injection of the vocal cords is a useful exercise in terminally ill patients as an improvement in their voice will significantly improve their morale.

A procedure that claims to have a greater success rate, in terms of better and more long-lasting voice production, is thyroplasty. This can be performed under local anaesthetic and sedation. A window is cut in the thyroid cartilage and a piece of preshaped silastic inserted in the paraglottic space; the position of the medialised cord can be checked using the nasendoscope and minor adjustments made depending upon the position of the cord. The patient can be asked to phonate and cough so that an accurate assessment of the voice can be made perioperatively. This procedure maintains the integrity of the mucosal wave on the vocal fold, which leads to a higher quality voice.

Some patients with a bilateral vocal cord palsy after total thyroidectomy may survive for many years without problems. A severe cold may, however, cause critical narrowing of the glottis and stridor. Such patients have good voice but poor exercise tolerance. The two surgical options are to bypass the larynx with a tracheostomy or to perform an arytenoidectomy to enlarge the glottic airway – this is usually carried out with a laser to help haemostasis. This procedure leads to a better airway but a much worse voice and many patients prefer a tracheostomy with a speaking valve to maintain near-normal voice.

PHARYNGEAL FOREIGN BODIES

Foreign bodies in the pharynx form a large part of an otolaryngologist's emergency workload. Foreign bodies may be accidentally ingested (for example coins, dentures and occasional oddities such as the pipe-stem shown in Fig. 29.4) or be related to the diet. Fishbones are commonly encountered as foreign bodies and the site of impaction is predictable: they may get stuck in the tonsil, and these are easily seen as fine strand-like protuberances that cause intense irritation. They are easily removed. Other common sites are the lingual tonsil, vallecula, pyriform fossa and cricopharyngeus. The history is crucial: some

fishbones are relatively radio-opaque and are easily confused with partially calcified sections of the thyroid cartilage. A pharyngoscopy may be performed on the basis of the history even if there is a negative X-ray. There is often the sensation of a foreign body that persists for days. This is usually the result of a scratch of the pharyngeal mucosa and all that is required is reassurance that there is no foreign body present.

The other common cause of foreign body obstruction is a food bolus. This is usually meat that has been bolted or not adequately chewed, often in patients with ill-fitting dentures. Patients present soon after ingestion with absolute dysphagia, incontinent of saliva and in considerable discomfort. A radiograph may not help but should nevertheless be performed to exclude cervical osteophytes that can complicate pharyngoscopy. The food may have become obstructed due to cricopharyngeal spasm and occasionally the bolus will pass spontaneously. Fizzy drinks may encourage passage and it is worth

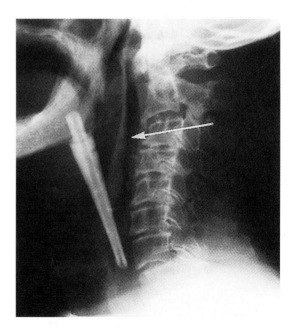

Fig. 29.4 A great variety of foreign bodies can impact in the pharynx: fish bones and meat bones are common. A pipe-stem is somewhat unusual, but note how air is present due to perforation into the retropharyngeal space (arrowed).

trying a dose of a smooth-muscle relaxant such as buscopan. If there is no success in a short space of time, however, the patient should undergo pharyngo-oesophagoscopy to remove the bolus. Delay is dangerous as peristalsis continues and can lead to perforation of the pharynx or oesophagus. If the bolus is stuck at mid- or lower oesophageal level it can be pushed through into the stomach using a flexible oesophagoscope (assuming there is no history of stricture). A nasogastric tube may need to be passed if removal has been traumatic.

GLOSSOPHARYNGEAL NEURALGIA

This is a condition similar to trigeminal neuralgia. Patients complain of brief, agonising, stabbing pains on one side of the neck, often precipitated by swallowing. There may be pain deep in the ear, and palpation of the tonsillar fossa may trigger the pain. Other causes of neuralgic pain, in particular skull base tumours, should be excluded. A long styloid process can mimic this condition and this can be seen on a radiograph.

Pain relief may be obtained with carbamazepine, but it is sometimes necessary to section the nerve. This can be performed through the tonsillar fossa, although it is occasionally necessary to divide it via a craniotomy.

MOTOR NEURONE DISEASE (BULBAR PALSY)

This is a disease of late middle age where there is progressive degeneration of the motor neurones with associated loss of function and wasting of skeletal muscles. Any muscles in the body may be affected and progressive dysphagia and dysarthria are not uncommon. The classical sign of the bulbar presentation is fasciculation and wasting of the tongue as a result of degeneration of the hypoglossal nuclei. Aspiration is the most dangerous complication; the subsequent pneumonia may be the patient's terminal illness. There is no treatment, other than supportive measures, for this relentless and distressing disease.

GLOBUS PHARYNGEUS

This disorder is commonly encountered in otolaryngology clinics. Patients, usually middle-aged women, are referred with a variety of symptoms, classically with a 'feeling of a lump in the throat'. The symptoms often start after a minor throat infection, and patients complain of an intermittent feeling of 'something stuck' behind the larynx or of a lump in the pharynx. This is always worse on swallowing saliva without food and there is no true dysphagia. The sensation is in the midline. It may be precipitated or worsened by a postnasal drip or reflux oesophagitis and these conditions should be excluded.

The differential diagnosis is a hypopharyngeal carcinoma, which itself may present with non-specific symptoms. Patients with the history described above, who have an intermittent rather than progressive problem and are non-smokers, are extremely unlikely to have a neoplastic lesion. Investigations should be kept to a minimum as these may enhance a patient's anxiety: positive reassurance that there is no serious pathology is usually sufficient. If not, a videofluoroscopy and even a pharyngoscopy may be necessary, mainly to reassure the patient – in the vast majority this is unnecessary. Reflux oesophagitis and nasal disease need to be treated appropriately.

PHARYNGEAL DIVERTICULAE (PHARYNGEAL POUCHES)

These are pulsion diverticulae through the posterior pharyngeal wall just above cricopharyngeus. The muscle wall is particularly weak here (Killian's dehiscence) and if there is persistent cricopharyngeal spasm or incoordination of cricopharyngeal relaxation, the intraluminal pressure in the pharynx rises and mucosa bulges posteriorly. Eventually a pouch of mucosa forms and lies posteriorly to the upper oesophagus (Fig. 29.5).

Food may collect in the pouch and cause dysphagia (which worsens as the pouch enlarges) and regurgitation of the contents into the mouth. An aspiration pneumonia can also develop. In large pouches, dysphagia may be nearly complete and the

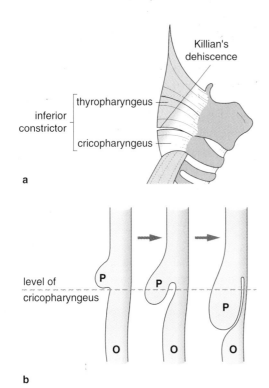

Fig. 29.5 (a) A pharyngeal diverticulum developing from Killian's dehiscence between the two portions of the inferior constrictor (thyropharyngeus and cricopharyngeus). (b) With time, the pouch (P) grows and the upper oesophagus (O), especially the entrance to it, is progressively compressed.

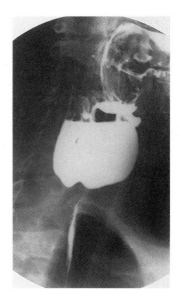

Fig. 29.6 A pharyngeal diverticulum demonstrated by a barium swallow examination.

patient may be wasted and very unwell. The diagnosis is made on barium swallow, which shows a large blind-ended sac behind a narrowed upper oesophagus. In cases of progressive dysphagia this investigation should always be performed before endoscopy; this is because an oesophagoscope will preferentially pass into the pouch, and, unless the surgeon is aware of the diagnosis, it is quite easy to perforate the tip of the pouch, causing a mediastinitis (Fig. 29.6). Treatment is surgical: the underlying pathology of cricopharyngeal spasm is dealt with by cricopharyngeal myotomy. The classic procedure is excision of the pouch and myotomy via an external incision, although an alternative is to divide the party wall between the pouch and oesophagus, creating one large cavity and performing a myotomy at the same time. An endoscopic stapling gun cuts the wall and securely staples the incised edges, preventing an oesophageal leak. It is a straightforward procedure: the patient can start eating soon afterwards and may be discharged 1–2 days postoperatively; this is quicker than the standard approach, an important consideration with frail patients. This is now generally felt to be the method of choice for treating pharyngeal pouches.

LARYNGOCELE

Laryngocele is a somewhat curious disorder which supposedly occurs mainly in players of wind instruments. It is essentially a pulsion diverticulum which forms from the ventricle of the larynx. For a time the swelling remains 'internal' in the larynx. There is a change in the quality of the voice and a smooth swelling may be seen in the lateral wall of the larynx. Eventually the diverticulum grows large enough to reach the exterior of the larynx between the superior and inferior constrictors and then forms an air-containing swelling in the neck. This is compressible and will enlarge with the Valsalva manoeuvre. Occasionally the lesion may become encysted and fluid-containing, and can then become infected and form an abscess. The clinician should be aware that a carcinoma of the laryngeal ventricle (which will be difficult to visualise) may rarely be associated with a laryngocele; all patients

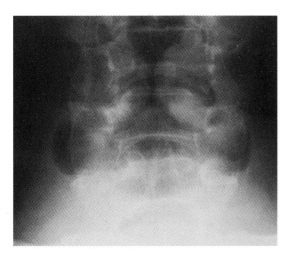

Fig. 29.7 Bilateral laryngoceles. The laryngocele is one of very few gas-containing swellings in the neck.

> ➤ **Key points**
>
> ➤ Inflammatory vocal cord lesions should be treated by a combination of vocal hygiene, voice therapy and surgery.
> ➤ Aspiration is a serious complication of sensory paralysis of the larynx.
> ➤ Vocal cord palsy may be caused by carcinoma of the bronchus.
> ➤ The site of obstruction of foreign bodies in the pharynx is predictable.
> ➤ Pharyngeal pouches are caused by cricopharyngeal incoordination and should be treated surgically.

with a laryngocele therefore need a microlaryngoscopy. If the lesion is troublesome it should be excised externally (Fig. 29.7).

Neoplastic disease of the larynx and pharynx

30

INTRODUCTION

Benign tumours of the larynx and pharynx are rare. Lipomas or fibromas may occasionally present with dysphagia in the upper aerodigestive tract; papillomas are essentially a disease of childhood and are dealt with in Chapter 28.

With the exception of lymphomas, which will be discussed later in the chapter, malignant tumours of the larynx and pharynx are almost exclusively squamous cell carcinomas. Adenocarcinomas and adenoid cystic carcinomas occur rarely, as do metastases. Most tumours in this region present late because of the clinically 'silent' areas from which they arise; the prognosis is therefore almost universally poor and this makes the choice of management options difficult. The exception to this is glottic carcinoma. This presents early, has a low incidence of metastatic lymphadenopathy and in a large proportion of patients the early tumours can be cured.

Aetiology

Apart from nasopharyngeal carcinoma (which will be discussed separately), all upper aerodigestive tract carcinomas have two principal aetiological factors in common: tobacco smoking and alcohol intake. The likelihood of a tumour developing is related to the quantity of tobacco smoked, and cessation of smoking leads to a decline in incidence of these tumours. Excessive alcohol intake, especially of spirits, acts synergistically with smoking to increase the incidence of tumours. It therefore follows that an education programme designed to stop people smoking at all, or drinking excessively will decrease the incidence of laryngeal and pharyngeal tumours and will improve prognosis in affected individuals.

Principles of treatment

The principles of treating malignant tumours in these areas are similar. They can be considered under the headings of definitive or palliative treatment.

Definitive treatment consists of radiotherapy or surgery, or a combination of modalities. When planning surgical treatment, consideration must be given to reconstructive techniques. In principle, early tumours are treated by single modality therapy (radiotherapy or surgery), while more advanced tumours are treated by combined surgery and radiotherapy. No overall advantage has been shown for chemotherapy in head and neck cancer apart from nasopharyngeal carcinoma. In general (although there are exceptions) patients who have nodal metastases are treated by primary surgery. Patients can be rehabilitated by judicious use of free and pedicled skin, muscle and bone flaps to reconstruct defects made by resection of tumours.

A large number of patients with these tumours are incurable at presentation. It is a difficult management challenge to identify such patients as they need to be palliated so they can live the remainder of their lives free of pain and with minimal morbidity. One-third of patients with oro- and hypopharyngeal tumours fall into this category.

TNM classification

It is helpful to stage tumours in order to decide – on the basis of published evidence – what the optimum treatment is for a particular neoplasm. It also means that results for the different stages of disease may be compared using a variety of treatment modalities and between different centres. The most common classification is the tumour, node, metastasis (TNM) system, in which account is taken of the local tumour status, whether there are nodal metastases and their extent, and whether there is any evidence of distant metastases. Each site in the head and neck has its own classification. When investigating tumours their topography should be annotated on a standardised map.

LARYNGEAL CARCINOMA

The larynx is the most common site for carcinoma in the upper aerodigestive tract, occurring in about 5 per 100 000 of the population. It is a disease of the middle-aged and elderly and is predominantly a disease affecting men rather than women. Interestingly, tumours of the supraglottis are more common in certain parts of the world (for example the Mediterranean countries) than in the UK, and the overall incidence varies widely throughout the world. Cigarette smoking is the most significant predisposing factor and alcohol intake (especially of spirits) acts synergistically with smoking; it must be remembered, however, that laryngeal cancer does occur in non-smokers.

For oncological purposes the larynx is divided into the supraglottis, glottis (vocal cords and arytenoids) and subglottis (Ch. 24). The presentation will be discussed below. Tumours of the vocal cord usually appear as raised, warty growths on one vocal cord, while supraglottic tumours tend to be exophytic or polypoid excrescences. Unilateral lesions must always be viewed with suspicion. Microscopically these tumours are almost exclusively squamous cell carcinomas, ranging from carcinoma in situ, where the basement membrane has not been breached, to poorly differentiated invasive carcinoma.

Spread of laryngeal carcinoma is influenced by the site of origin in the larynx. Metastasis takes place along well-defined pathways to lymph nodes of the jugular chain (levels II–IV) (Fig. 16.2) or to paratracheal nodes when there is subglottic extension. Direct spread occurs into the pre-epiglottic and paraglottic spaces; extension into the thyroid or cricoid cartilage carries a poor prognosis. The glottis fortunately has a very sparse lymphatic drainage so that lymphatic metastasis from glottic tumours is quite rare. This is an important prognostic factor and, combined with the fact that glottic tumours present earlier, means that these tumours tend to have a higher cure rate than supraglottic tumours of comparable stage. Early laryngeal cancer, especially of the glottis, carries a remarkably good prognosis. T1 glottic tumours (see below) carry a 5-year survival of approximately 90% when treated by primary radiotherapy.

Presentation

Progressive hoarseness (dysphonia) is the cardinal symptom of laryngeal carcinoma. Because even an early tumour of the glottis will interfere with the movement of the vocal cords, they present early compared to supraglottic and the exceedingly rare subglottic tumours. For this reason any patient over the age of 40 with a hoarse voice lasting more than 2 weeks should be referred for specialist assessment by indirect laryngoscopy. Younger patients, especially if smokers, should be referred after 3–4 weeks of hoarseness. Other symptoms usually indicate advanced disease and these include dyspnoea and stridor, dysphagia (indicating pharyngeal involvement) and pain. Pain in the ear (referred otalgia) is an ominous sign reflecting advanced disease.

Examination in the clinic revolves around laryngoscopy, either with a mirror or flexible nasolaryngoscope. Any asymmetry is noted and the extent of any lesion assessed (Fig. 30.1). Vocal cord mobility must be determined at this stage: it may be normal or reduced or the cord may be paralysed; this information is important for staging. The neck is examined for metastatic lymphadenopathy. If any abnormality is detected a chest radiograph should be arranged.

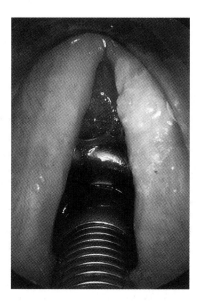

Fig. 30.1 T1 glottic tumour of the right vocal cord.

Management

This begins with the diagnosis. Patients undergo a microlaryngoscopy under general anaesthetic, during which the entire larynx and pharynx is assessed and the neck and tongue base palpated. The lesion is examined carefully and palpated gently to assess depth of invasion and extent. Biopsies are then taken and the extent of the tumour is annotated on a standardised diagram. A clinical TNM staging is now possible. Box 30.1 illustrates the T staging of glottic tumours, which are the most common

---

■ **Box 30.1**

T staging of glottic carcinoma

- ■ T1a   Tumour confined to one vocal cord, normal mobility
- ■ T1b   Tumour on both vocal cords, normal mobility
- ■ T2   Tumour limited to one vocal cord, reduced mobility and/or extends to supra- or subglottis
- ■ T3   Tumour limited to larynx with vocal cord fixation
- ■ T4   Tumour extends beyond larynx (e.g. to pharynx, thyroid cartilage)

---

encountered. For staging of nodal disease see Chapter 18.

Treatment depends upon the T stage as well as patient preference. The standard treatment for T1 and T2 tumours of the supraglottis and glottis is radical radiotherapy, which produces excellent results, especially for glottic tumours. T4 tumours should be treated by total laryngectomy and post-operative radiotherapy. There is still some debate about the optimum treatment for T3 tumours; supraglottic tumours should be treated by laryngectomy, as should those glottic tumours with bulky disease. Some patients can be cured with radical radiotherapy, retaining an intact larynx, although the voice may not be very good. Salvage laryngectomy following failed radiotherapy gives acceptable survival results, although the postoperative morbidity is higher.

Laryngectomy

Removal of the larynx is a radical procedure with severe consequences for subsequent communication; it is undoubtedly an effective operation, however, for controlling laryngeal cancer and is indicated for advanced and recurrent disease. Partial laryngectomy is occasionally indicated for smaller tumours. Total laryngectomy also involves creation of an opening into the pharynx and this needs to be reconstituted. Good surgical technique combined with surgical voice reconstruction (see below) produces normal swallowing and adequate speech for communication, with no risk of aspiration. Patients' quality of life is usually surprisingly good (Figs 30.2 and 30.3).

Management of stridor: tracheostomy

Patients with advanced tumours, or exophytic glottic tumours, may present with inspiratory stridor. This is an extremely dangerous symptom as it implies impending airway obstruction and urgent and radical procedures are necessary to secure it. Certain diseases that present with stridor, such as supraglottitis, can usually be managed successfully by medical means, with intravenous corticosteroids and antibiotics (Ch. 27); however, malignant tumours of the larynx and pharynx that present with stridor need

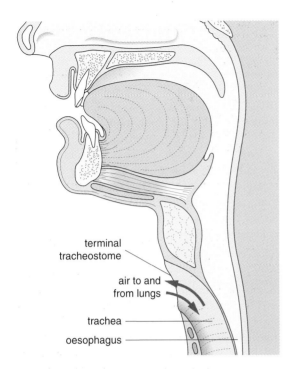

terminal
tracheostome

air to and
from lungs

trachea

oesophagus

Fig. 30.2 Following laryngectomy the trachea terminates as a stoma above the suprasternal notch.

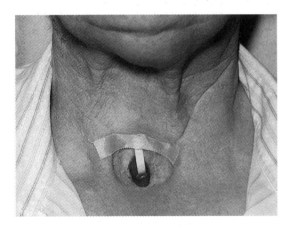

Fig. 30.3 Tracheal stoma in patient who has undergone a laryngectomy (such a patient is known as a 'laryngectomee'). A Blom Singer speaking valve is in place.

to be managed by a temporary tracheostomy. There are other indications for tracheostomy and these are listed in Box 30.2.

Tracheostomy may be performed by an open or percutaneous technique. The latter is increasingly

---

■ **Box 30.2**

Indications for tracheostomy

■ Respiratory distress (stridor)
- Malignant tumours of larynx and pharynx
- Infective
    supraglottitis
    neck space abscesses
- Bilateral vocal cord palsy
■ Radical neck surgery
- Perioperatively to protect airway
- Major oral and pharyngeal surgery
■ Reduce secretions
- To protect airway from aspiration
    partial laryngeal and pharyngeal surgery
    neurological disease, e.g. motor neurone
    disease
■ Reduce dead space
- Patients on intensive care requiring
    prolonged ventilation

---

used in intensive care situations and when an elective tracheostomy is performed perioperatively; it does not have a place in the emergency situation and every otolaryngologist should be competent to perform an open tracheostomy.

In cases of stridor where the security of the airway is in doubt, the operation is performed under local anaesthesia. The patient may need to be sitting up slightly, but the neck should be extended as much as possible. After the infiltration of local anaesthetic, a horizontal incision centred on the midline is made, halfway between the cricoid and suprasternal notch. The platysma is divided and the guiding principle is then to dissect in the midline. The strap muscles are retracted laterally and the thyroid isthmus is encountered: this is divided and transfixed. The cricoid and trachea are identified. At this stage the tracheostomy tube is checked, the cuff inflated to ascertain that it is intact, and the connections to the anaesthetic apparatus are also checked. A window is cut in the trachea below the second ring and the cuffed tube is inserted. A general anaesthetic is given at this point so that the tumour may be assessed.

Postoperatively the patient has to be nursed carefully, with judicious use of suction; the tracheostomy should be humidified to prevent excessive crusting. The cuff can be deflated to allow the patient to speak around the tube. Once the tract is established, a small uncuffed tube with an inner tube is inserted; this allows for the tube to be cleaned without removing it in its entirety.

The most worrying complication is if the tube falls out or is dislodged. Expert nursing is required and facilities should be at hand to allow rapid and safe reinsertion. The first tracheostomy change should be done by the surgeon who performed the operation, and Box 30.3 lists the equipment needed by a patient's bedside for a tube change.

Closure of a tracheostomy is easy when indicated. The tube is simply removed and an occlusive dressing applied to the site. The track usually closes in a matter of hours or at most a few days.

Rehabilitation

The most devastating consequence of total laryngectomy is the loss of the voice, and thus the means of communicating with others (Box 30.4). In the vast majority of patients, however, a satisfactory voice can be achieved postoperatively. Traditionally

■ Box 30.3

Tracheostomy change

- Equipment
  - Suction
  - Good lighting (head light)
  - Tracheal dilators
  - Replacement tube
- Procedure for tube change
  - Expert nursing assistance
  - Patient sitting up
  - Suction before removing tube
  - Prepare tube, check cuff if necessary
  - Check equipment to hand
  - Explain procedure to patient
  - Change tube
  - Check correct position

■ Box 30.4

Methods of communication after laryngectomy

- Pen and paper
- Silent articulation
- Electric larynx
- Oesophageal speech
- Tracheo-oesophageal speech (surgical voice restoration)

patients have been taught oesophageal speech: they learn to swallow air and expel it in short gulps, causing the pharynx to vibrate, thus producing sound. In a small minority excellent voice can be achieved, and about one-third of laryngectomees produce satisfactory voice by this method. For those unable to achieve oesophageal speech an electronic vibrator may be applied to the neck. This causes the airway to vibrate and thus produce sound; the voice is usually of very poor quality, however, and difficult to understand.

In the last 15 years the concept of surgical voice restoration has been developed. This utilises a one-way valve that is inserted in a fistula created between the posterior tracheal wall and the oesophagus. The valve prevents aspiration and allows air to be diverted from the lungs into the pharynx. The neopharynx then vibrates, producing sound that is converted into recognisable speech by the articulators of the mouth. The advantage of using the lungs as a reservoir is that an increased volume of air and increased power are available to generate the voice. The tracheo-oesophageal puncture is now usually performed at laryngectomy as a primary procedure, and the valve is fitted within 2 weeks of surgery. Satisfactory speech can be achieved in over 80% of laryngectomees. Different valves may be used to suit different patients. Figure 30.4 illustrates a 'duckbill' Blom Singer valve, which the patient is taught to remove, clean and replace. Indwelling valves are an alternative. A valve in situ in a laryngectomee is seen in Figure 30.3. This procedure has revolutionised the quality of life of many laryngectomees.

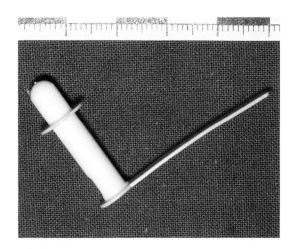

Fig. 30.4 A Blom Singer speaking valve. The thick cylindrical portion passes through the surgically created tracheo-oesophageal fistula. The thin flange is taped to the skin above the tracheal stoma (see Fig. 30.3).

TUMOURS OF THE PHARYNX

Nasopharynx

Nasopharyngeal carcinoma (NPC) differs from other malignancies of the head and neck in many ways. It is not clearly related to smoking and alcohol, has a marked racial diversity and occurs at a younger age.

This tumour is found particularly in southern Chinese populations and is the most common carcinoma occurring in Hong Kong males under 50 years of age. It is quite uncommon in white populations, but Chinese people who move to Western countries retain the high incidence, suggesting a genetic predisposition. There is strong evidence that a high intake of salted fish containing nitrosamines acts as a promoter in carcinogenesis. Infection with Epstein–Barr virus in genetically susceptible individuals promotes development of NPC. Monitoring levels of viral antigen has a role in screening susceptible individuals and as a marker for recurrent disease.

NPC occurs as a space-occupying lesion in the nasopharynx arising from the junction of the nasal cavity and nasopharynx, often in the region of the fossa of Rosenmuller. In endemic areas undifferentiated carcinoma is the most common histological type, while in sporadic cases, such as occur in Europe, well-differentiated tumours are more common. NPC has a high propensity for lymphatic metastasis, initially to the retropharyngeal nodes and then to neck nodes, classically in the posterior triangle and often bilaterally. If diagnosed early the prognosis is good, but unfortunately most tumours are diagnosed when advanced, because of their clinically silent nature, making the prognosis much worse. Only 10% of tumours are diagnosed at an early stage.

Symptoms and signs at presentation include painless, enlarged lymph nodes in the neck (present in approximately 75% of patients at presentation), nasal obstruction, epistaxis, diminished hearing and tinnitus caused by otitis media with effusion, cranial nerve dysfunction, sore throat and headache. The nasopharynx is a common site for an occult primary in the presence of malignant cervical lymphadenopathy (Ch. 17).

In the absence of a ready explanation for these symptoms, NPC should be excluded. Adults with a persistent unilateral middle ear effusion must have a biopsy of the postnasal space. Similarly, patients with a malignant neck lump and an unknown primary should have their postnasal space examined and biopsied.

Treatment of NPC is by radical radiotherapy to the primary site and the neck (because of the high incidence of lymphatic metastases). NPC can be a very radiosensitive tumour. Adjuvant chemotherapy has been used with some success in comparison to other head and neck malignancies. Surgery is reserved for salvage neck dissection in those patients with persistent or recurrent neck disease following radiotherapy.

The radiotherapy fields used are wide and include a large proportion of the oral cavity. Side-effects of radiotherapy are common and can be severe. One of the most common complications is marked xerostomia, which is very unpleasant for the patient and can contribute to dental caries. Otological and neurological complications may also ensue.

Oropharynx

The most common malignant tumour of the oropharynx is squamous cell carcinoma; however, lymphoma is not unusual (comprising 25% of malignant oropharyngeal tumours) because of the large amount of lymphoid tissue in the oropharynx. Biopsy of malignant-looking tissue is essential even before palliative treatment because lymphoma generally has a better prognosis than squamous carcinoma. (For a more detailed description of lymphoma see below). Minor salivary gland tumours are rare.

Oropharyngeal carcinoma is a rare tumour occurring most commonly in the seventh decade of life and being much more prevalent in males. As in almost all head and neck tumours, smoking and alcohol consumption predispose to the development of these tumours. They occur most often in the tonsil, being found (in decreasing order of frequency) in the tongue base, soft palate, vallecula and posterior pharyngeal wall. A unilaterally enlarged tonsil in an adult, especially with known risk factors, is an absolute indication for tonsillectomy. Squamous carcinomas at this site are generally ulcerated, while lymphomas appear more bulky and fleshy. These tumours are classified as well differentiated, moderately differentiated or poorly differentiated and this classification has a bearing upon the prognosis.

Because of the plentiful lymphatic supply, lymph node metastasis is quite common. Even if no lymph node is palpable there is still a high incidence of occult metastases and this has an influence on prognosis and management. Bilateral metastases may occur, especially in midline tumours. The spread to lymph node groups is predictable, most spreading to level II nodes initially. The prognosis of oropharyngeal cancer is poor, partly because of the late presentation of the primary and partly owing to the ready propensity to lymph node spread.

Tumours at this site often remain silent until they are quite advanced. Presenting symptoms include sore throat, pain on swallowing, dysphagia and referred otalgia (an ominous sign). Ten per cent of patients present with a lump in the neck.

Examination usually reveals an ulcerated or exophytic tumour; assessment is made of the oral cavity (including dental status and hypoglossal nerve function), larynx and pharynx and neck. A chest X-ray is requested and a fine-needle aspiration cytology specimen taken of any neck nodes.

The next step in assessment is a panendoscopy. Biopsies are taken (in the form of tonsillectomy if the site is the tonsil). If lymphoma is suspected, part of the biopsy should be sent fresh to the pathology laboratory so that special staining can be performed. MRI is the best modality for assessing extension into the tongue; an isotope bone scan may be necessary to assess mandibular invasion. The tumour can then be staged according to the TNM system.

Some patients are incurable and should be offered palliative treatment. Major surgical procedures are occasionally justified as a palliative procedure to relieve pain and dysphagia.

Curative treatment for squamous cell carcinoma is either by radical radiotherapy or surgery, which is usually combined with postoperative adjuvant radiotherapy. In principle, small tumours with no palpable lymph node metastases are treated with radical radiotherapy, while patients who have palpable metastases are treated with surgery. Because of the high incidence of lymphatic metastasis, the neck is generally treated – either by radiotherapy or by an elective, selective neck dissection. Tonsillar tumours without palpable lymphatic metastases respond well to radiotherapy and have a good prognosis.

Surgery for oropharyngeal carcinoma is a major undertaking and requires careful planning in terms of method of resection and technique for reconstruction. Access is difficult and is usually via a mandibulotomy. Resection has to be oncologically sound, while preserving as much tissue as possible for function. New techniques for reconstruction have improved functional outcome. Defects may be repaired using a myocutaneous flap (for example the pectoralis major flap, which provides bulk for defects) or free flaps where a microvascular reconstruction technique is applied. The most common flap employed is the radial forearm free flap which is pliable and gives good postoperative function.

Bone for mandibular reconstruction can also be brought in as a composite free flap with skin and muscle. Patients need a perioperative tracheostomy and will require enteral feeding (for example via a percutaneous gastrostomy) while their swallowing is rehabilitated postoperatively.

Management of oropharyngeal cancer is a good example of a situation in which cooperation between different disciplines is essential. Specialists in the field of resection, reconstruction, clinical oncology and palliative medicine need to be consulted to arrive at the optimum treatment plan tailored to an individual's unique circumstances.

Hypopharynx

The three sites in which hypopharyngeal carcinomas appear are the pyriform fossa, postcricoid region and posterior pharyngeal wall (in decreasing order of frequency). Hypopharyngeal tumours present particular problems in management because of their proximity to the larynx. Hypopharyngeal carcinoma is a rare disease in the UK. There are national and regional variations in the relative frequency of occurrence of pyriform fossa and postcricoid lesions, the latter being more common in India and in England and Wales. While pyriform fossa tumours are more common in males, the sex incidence is reversed for postcricoid tumours, which are more prevalent in females. It is a smoking-related disease and the effect of alcohol is synergistic. Previous ionising radiation to the thyroid gland is also a predisposing factor.

Paterson–Brown Kelly syndrome (Plummer–Vinson syndrome) is a premalignant condition occurring in middle-aged females. It is characterised by a microcytic, hypochromic anaemia, koilonychia, angular stomatitis and glossitis and dysphagia caused by a postcricoid web. The incidence of this syndrome has fallen sharply as a result of improved nutrition. Approximately one-quarter of patients with Paterson–Brown Kelly syndrome develop postcricoid carcinoma, often decades later. These patients need to have their anaemia corrected and should be followed up for life, with biopsy of any webs demonstrated on barium swallow.

Hypopharyngeal tumours may be exophytic or ulcerative; on indirect laryngoscopy a pyriform fossa tumour may be seen as a cauliflower-shaped excrescence appearing lateral to the larynx. They are almost exclusively squamous cell carcinomas of varying differentiation.

The hypopharynx has a rich lymphatic supply, making lymphatic metastases common, especially from pyriform fossa lesions. Bilateral spread is usual from all sites. Postcricoid tumours may spread down the oesophagus by skip lesions and posterior pharyngeal wall tumours can spread directly into prevertebral muscles. The prognosis of these tumours is universally poor. One-third are incurable at presentation: the presence of lymphatic metastases reduces the 5-year survival by at least 50%.

Box 30.5 shows the clinical presentation of hypopharyngeal carcinoma. Progressive dysphagia for solids, then liquids, is the cardinal symptom and must be distinguished from the more vague 'feeling of a lump' in globus pharyngeus.

Examination may reveal a neck mass and loss of laryngeal crepitus. Indirect laryngoscopy is often normal but most tumours are advanced at presentation, so a pyriform fossa mass, salivary pooling or associated laryngeal involvement (for example vocal cord palsy) may all be seen.

Investigation is directed at assessing the extent of the primary tumour, whether or not there is another tumour in the oesophagus or elsewhere (synchronous primary) and the status of the lymph nodes. A chest X-ray and barium swallow are essential and CT or MRI is usually indicated to assess the primary tumour and neck.

■ Box 30.5

Presentation of hypopharyngeal carcinoma

- Pain, usually lateralised, may radiate to the ear
- Dysphagia, usually constant, beware food 'sticking' on swallowing
- Haemoptysis
- Hoarseness, suggests extension to larynx
- Neck mass, may be direct extension or metastasis
- Weight loss

Treatment depends upon the stage. A few early tumours may be cured by radical radiotherapy; however, most are advanced at presentation and require surgery and postoperative adjuvant radiotherapy. It is unusual to be able to spare the larynx because it is usually involved in tumour. Postcricoid tumours are treated by a total pharyngolaryngectomy with a free jejunal interposition graft; if the oesophagus is involved in the chest, oesophagectomy is also required, with a stomach pull-up through the chest for reconstruction. Total pharyngolaryngectomy is usually preferable for pyriform fossa lesions; it is unwise to leave too small a pharyngeal remnant as postoperative pharyngeal strictures are a difficult problem to deal with. Both sides of the neck are usually treated by a radical or selective neck dissection.

Patient selection is important. These operations are major undertakings and the chance of cure has to be weighed up against quality of life; an elderly patient may not tolerate such a major procedure and palliative treatment may be more appropriate. This would consist of radiotherapy, analgesia and perhaps a gastrostomy.

LYMPHOMA OF THE HEAD AND NECK

Lymphoma is increasing in incidence. Because of the large amount of lymphatic tissue in the head and neck, disease in this region is not uncommon.

Lymphoma may be nodal or extranodal; it is traditionally classified as Hodgkin's or non-Hodgkin's lymphoma, depending upon the presence or absence of Reed–Sternberg cells. Further classification is important for treatment and prognostic purposes and is now largely based on immunohistological techniques. This is beyond the scope of this book but it must be remembered that, when taking a biopsy of a lesion that is likely to be a lymphoma, some of it should be sent immediately to the laboratory as the immunological characteristics are best defined on fresh specimens. Lymphoma characteristically presents in the neck as multiple, small to medium-sized rubbery lymph nodes on one or both sides of the neck. There may also be axillary or inguinal lymphadenopathy. The patient is generally younger than is usual for squamous cell carcinoma, and may experience weight loss and night sweats if the disease is generalised.

Extranodal disease carries a poorer prognosis than nodal disease. It may occur anywhere in the region but is most common in the tonsil and tongue base. These lesions distinguish themselves from squamous cell carcinoma by being bulky, fleshy non-ulcerated tumours.

The otolaryngologist should confine himself to performing a biopsy and then refer the patient to a specialist in lymphoma management for staging and treatment. Investigations include whole body CT, haematological and serological tests and bone marrow sampling. Treatment of localised disease is by radical radiotherapy, and by chemotherapy if the lymphoma is more widespread. Depending upon the tumour classification, results of treatment can be dramatically successful even for large tumours.

> **Key points**
> ➤ Every effort must be made to produce an accurate TNM staging on every tumour.
> ➤ Patients with a persistently hoarse voice need examining to exclude laryngeal carcinoma.
> ➤ A unilaterally enlarged tonsil in an adult is an absolute indication for tonsillectomy to exclude malignancy.
> ➤ Persistent, unilateral otitis media with effusion in an adult is an absolute indication for postnasal space biopsy to exclude nasopharyngeal carcinoma.
> ➤ The incidence of lymphatic metastases is high in many head and neck tumours and the neck usually has to be included in the treatment plan.
> ➤ Making the correct treatment choice for each patient is difficult and requires multidisciplinary consultation.

Oesophagus

FOREIGN BODIES

Food boluses are the most common foreign bodies to obstruct the oesophagus. The site is usually at one of the points of constriction in the oesophagus (Ch. 24). They may be secondary to a benign or malignant stricture so it is imperative to obtain a good history. Progressive dysphagia prior to the acute event suggests an underlying mechanical problem. As with pharyngeal foreign bodies (Ch. 29), administration of a muscle relaxant such as buscopan may allow the muscle to relax sufficiently to enable the bolus to pass spontaneously. If it does not, oesophagoscopy should be undertaken. Rigid oesophagoscopy is a dangerous procedure with the very real risk of oesophageal perforation. The oesophagus should be treated as if the wall were made of wet blotting paper. The patient should be given a good muscle relaxant and the lumen kept in view at all times. Postoperatively, the signs of perforation that should be watched for are sharp interscapular pain, increased respiratory rate and pyrexia: these patients should be promptly referred to a thoracic unit for further management. For distal oesophageal problems, flexible oesophagoscopy is a safer and equally effective procedure. The bolus can be pushed into the stomach, where it will cease to cause any further symptoms.

In cases where a foreign body has impacted above a stricture the bolus needs to be removed and the stricture biopsied, followed by gentle dilatation under direct vision. Figure 31.1 shows a modern oesophagoscope, and Figure 31.2 gum elastic bougies for dilating strictures.

GASTRO-OESOPHAGEAL REFLUX

Gastro-oesophageal reflux (GOR) has been implicated in the aetiology of many otolaryngological conditions, although this is on the basis of very little hard evidence. GOR can present to the otolaryngologist with symptoms in the pharynx and larynx such as heartburn and waterbrash; a

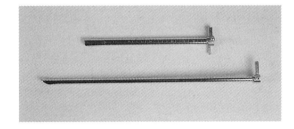

Fig. 31.1 Modern rigid oesophagoscope.

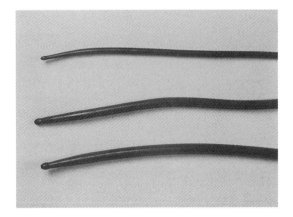

Fig. 31.2 Oesophageal bougies for dilating an oesophageal stricture.

Oesophagus

stricture resulting from severe prolonged GOR may be a cause of dysphagia or food bolus obstruction. It is thought that globus pharyngeus may be secondary to GOR, although this is not proven. It may exacerbate the condition, as does postnasal drip, but is not the cause.

A link has been established between GOR and asthma in adults and children, and other laryngeal diseases such as contact ulcers are thought to be associated with inflammation of the laryngeal mucosa by acidic stomach contents. Other factors such as poor vocalisation and smoking are more important causes.

A definite diagnosis of GOR can only be made by a complex process of ambulatory 24-hour pH monitoring. Treatment is by weight loss and cessation of smoking; if medication is indicated and reflux proven, a proton pump inhibitor such as omeprazole may be prescribed.

CARCINOMA

Oesophageal carcinoma (Fig. 31.3) may present to the otolaryngologist in a variety of ways. Food bolus obstruction may be the first presenting feature of this tumour or the patient may be referred to the ENT clinic for an assessment of dysphagia. In the history the dysphagia is felt at a lower level than in pharyngeal lesions. Patients with extraluminal spread of oesophageal carcinoma may present with or develop a hoarse voice caused by a recurrent laryngeal nerve palsy.

Oesophageal carcinoma is a relatively common tumour compared to most head and neck cancers. It is a disease of the elderly and has a strong geographical distribution, being common in certain areas of France and South Africa. Smoking and excess alcohol intake are predisposing factors and tumours may be found throughout the oesophagus, being most common in the lower third. These are generally adenocarcinomas, while higher lesions are more commonly squamous cell carcinomas.

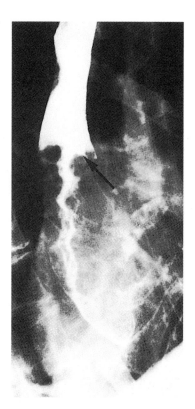

Fig. 31.3 Contrast radiograph showing carcinoma of the oesophagus. Note the irregularity of outline, particularly the upper edge (arrow).

Patients have a poor prognosis as they often present at an advanced stage. Palliative treatment may involve intubation, laser debulking or radiotherapy. Curative treatment depends upon stage and co-morbidity and involves either oesophagectomy or radiotherapy.

> ➤ **Key points**
>
> ➤ Complications of oesophagoscopy may be life threatening.
> ➤ Gastro-oesophageal reflux may produce a variety of throat/pharyngeal symptoms.

Index